Readers love The Power of Hope

'If ever there was a definition of hope, it was and is Kate Garraway! Kate Garraway's account of her husband's awful struggle with Covid is an incredible family love story that tears at your heart.'

'Very well written, very informative, at times heart rending, but an absolute must read!'

'The strength, determination, hope and love for Derek all shine through in this book.'

'A selfless and poignant story.'

'The highs and lows are written from the heart with the will to never give up hope.'

'This book is a truly amazing story of a family's love and strength through adversity.'

'A fantastic read. Could not put it down. A tale of love, courage and immense hope.'

'Kate was extremely honest throughout and brings home to so many what the pandemic has put us through. A worthy read.'

'Such a powerful story of being strong and not giving up.'

'Very honest and heartfelt.'

'Amazing story of human survival and strength.'

'A beautiful book about hope in the most difficult of times.'

'A true story of never giving up. Miraculously narrated. A true inspiration.'

'Gripped to every page of this book, from beginning to end. Excellently written and by such a strong individual.'

'Everyone should read this wonderfully heartfelt inspiring book of love, hope and strength.'

Kate Garraway

The Power *of* Hope

**A STORY OF LOVE, FEAR AND
NEVER GIVING UP**

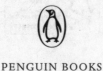

PENGUIN BOOKS

TRANSWORLD PUBLISHERS
Penguin Random House, One Embassy Gardens,
8 Viaduct Gardens, London SW11 7BW
www.penguin.co.uk

Transworld is part of the Penguin Random House group of companies
whose addresses can be found at global.penguinrandomhouse.com

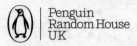

Penguin
Random House
UK

First published in Great Britain in 2021 by Bantam Press
an imprint of Transworld Publishers
Penguin paperback edition published 2022

A CIP catalogue record for this book
is available from the British Library.

ISBN 9780552178372

Typeset in Adobe Caslon by www.envyltd.co.uk
Printed and bound in Great Britain by Clays Ltd, Elcograf S.p.A.

The authorized representative in the EEA is Penguin Random House Ireland,
Morrison Chambers, 32 Nassau Street, Dublin D02 YH68.

Penguin Random House is committed to a sustainable
future for our business, our readers and our planet. This book
is made from Forest Stewardship Council® certified paper.

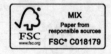

For Derek
And for everyone battling on through

Contents

Contents

Hope is not the conviction that something
will turn out well but the certainty that something
makes sense, regardless of how it turns out

Vaclav Havel

Prologue

Two years ago, none of us was prepared for the corona-virus pandemic: how could we have been? Even world-class experts were confounded by this unknown virus and its consequences for our bodies, our lives, our livelihoods. No one has escaped its effect. Like a tornado, it sucked in families, businesses and even governments, upending every aspect of our lives.

For months, we stood like *The Wizard of Oz*'s Dorothy, praying that the storm would pass, watching the wreckage of our former lives drop down from the sky and wondering when the spinning would come to an end. For the best part of a year, we have hung on to the thought that there still might be a clear threshold, a moment when it was over, when we could step over the line and things would finally be back to normal. These days I think we all have a sense that we're 'not in Kansas any more'. Nearly two years on, it seems clearer than ever that our lives have changed for ever.

The virus transformed my family, my marriage and my sense of self. I shared much of that change with you on *Good Morning Britain* and on Smooth Radio, and maybe you saw my documentary *Finding Derek*. But there was just as much change taking place in intensely private moments: the twitch of a finger, the flicker of an eye, the spark of hope kept alive in the small hours. And it's these moments I wanted to share with you in this book.

Each of us now has our Covid story to tell, and many of yours have helped me through some of the darkest nights and lowest points – especially since this book was first published last year. I will never be able to thank you enough for all the love and kindness you have shown me and my family. And I hope that in sharing our story with you, you may find some comfort in knowing that you haven't been alone, that none of us has. Because although this has undoubtedly been the hardest couple of years, for myself and my family, and for so many of you, it has also taught me an enormous amount about how much good is out there. And the true power of hope.

Today, I believe more than ever that hope is the incredible force that can get us through, and that it is all around us, solid as a rock, if we just know how to find it. Like Dorothy, who finds out in the end that she didn't need the Wizard of Oz after all, we all have the ability to help ourselves. Dorothy turned out to have what she needed to get herself home, if she just clicked her heels and felt it. And each of us has inside us the trick to make the magic of hope work for us.

This has been a big change for me. I don't think I understood hope at all before 2020, even though I used the word all the time.

'Are you going to be able to make it tonight?'

'Hope so!'

'You'll be brilliant at this! You have nothing to worry about!'

'Hope so!'

'Everything will work out in the end, you'll see.'

'Hope so!'

I used it almost like an apology in advance, a managing of expectations, when I didn't have the confidence that I could actually deliver anything I was 'hoping' for. I'd feel the urge to put it in when I couldn't be sure something was going to happen, when I wasn't confident something could be achieved, when there were no concrete facts available. For me, it was a 'try' word – a genuine longing, yes, but a wish rather than a solid promise. I realize now that that is, in fact, the opposite of how hope works. As soon as you wish for something, long for it, use hope as anything less than a certain belief, it drives the magic of hope further from you. I know this all sounds very hippie, but don't let that put you off. Two years ago, I would have had little faith in it too. My working life has been built on facts, on evidence, on holding people to account if they couldn't deliver their promises. And I relied on facts for my coping strategies in my personal life, too. Whenever something went wrong, or didn't go as I wanted, I would always try to find out how I could change it, trying to learn everything I could to improve, drawing on my experience of the past, using the evidence of my life to form a plan for the future to see me through to whatever goal I wanted to achieve.

There's nothing wrong with this, and it's something I continued to do throughout the very worst of this terrible period, and still do. And in many ways, it has paid off. After all, these days Derek *is* back at home, which is something we were not sure would ever be able to happen – even as I wrote the original edition of this book.

But it's not the whole picture. The trouble with what we have all been through during the Covid pandemic is that at every stage we couldn't be truly confident of the so-called facts. There has been precious little evidence from our past life experience on which to build a confident plan. At every stage, confusion and uncertainty have undermined us. We have seen this in our politicians, sometimes seemingly brimming with bullish spirit about what they know, and the next minute upended by new information, dramatically changing their previous operating tactics, with their ability to inspire trust left in tatters. We have seen it, too, in the brilliant scientists, having constantly to adjust their advice and their approach as Covid overturned what had previously been considered certain. It's been there in our medical professionals, fighting a war against a disease that defies their experience and their previous practice. We have been living with crippling uncertainty for weeks, then months and years, and I think we now know that we will have to live with it for many years to come.

We need something extra, some special magic ... and that magic is hope. That terrifying uncertainty.

In my personal Covid story, the uncertainty has been hardest to bear when I have seen it up close in our wonderful medical professionals. When the doctors could give me no guarantees as to whether Derek would live or die, whether he could hang on even for another hour or would slip away like so many thousands of other poor souls, I felt fear might crush me, consume me, drown me. Even now, with the medics still unable to confirm how or when Derek might recover further, there are days when the endless not-knowing gnaws me to the bone.

How could I find hope when the health professionals, the people I trusted most to deliver my biggest wish for Derek to survive, were left confounded? But as I struggled to stay afloat in this ocean of fear, I saw something even more powerful than medical facts and professional experience. It was the determination of doctors, nurses and other NHS workers to keep going against all the odds, in the face of exhaustion, even putting their own safety at risk. They never gave up hope, in spite of everything they were faced with. It was their hope that drove them forward, their certain belief that the war could be won, despite all the evidence of their eyes to the contrary. This drove them to learn quickly, to adapt and to invent new ways of working, to bring us a portfolio of vaccines in record time, to fight on to a better future. Hasn't that spirit always driven the medical and caring professions? Until Covid brought a new awareness of their uncertainty to us, we had been able to fool ourselves that they knew everything. Now we have to accept that the experts aren't always all-knowing, aren't always all-confident.

But we can truly believe in their spirit, their hope.

Once I managed to see this, even for a moment, I could allow true hope to come to me in all forms – from friends, family, strangers and experts – and discover new ways to move forward, to find a life raft.

I don't want you to think that I believe I now have all the answers – far from it. As you read on, you will see I have been honest about my failings and the darkest moments when they have crashed over me. I also know that I'm luckier than many others. I have so much to be grateful for, not least that Derek is still alive, and that we have already enjoyed nearly a year of him living back home with us. This, I know, has been denied to so many others. I'm grateful, too, for all the support that has surrounded me and how much I have learnt from others. One of my main reasons for writing this book was so I could share what has helped me. Even if I haven't quite mastered many of the techniques that have been suggested to me to make hope real, they might trigger something in you to help you face your own demons and whatever life chucks at you as the ripple effect of the pandemic continues to spread.

In this book, I have tried to be open and honest about all that we as a family have been through, and you will hear from many people who have shared our journey. But I'm painfully aware that one voice is still sadly absent: that of Derek. I know he would have wanted to tell his own story if he could – and one day he still may. In these pages, I have tried to do him – and all those who love him – justice, and his love and life are present in every line. I also know that he now draws great strength from the idea that what he has been through might help others. The brilliant team of doctors and specialists who have been looking after him have already learnt a huge amount from how this grim virus has affected him physically, and this in turn has gone on to help the treatment of others. On an emotional level, I hope that you will also draw something from how we, his family, have struggled to cope.

Thank you to everyone who has kept me going: you are all part of that positive energy. It has helped me to understand what hope is, and how we can put it to the best possible use. It is my wish that, in describing this journey, you might draw strength from hope, no matter what your circumstances. After all, in a world where so much that we thought was certain has changed in a heartbeat, I think it might be the most solid superpower we have.

Chapter 1

Beginnings

'This is going to be your year!' said Derek, as 31 December faded into 2020. As we raised a glass to each other at midnight, he announced with a flourish, 'Move over, Ant and Dec! You're not winning TV Personality of the Year in 2020 – my Kate is!' and promptly followed up with, 'Mind you, if you become a big star, you're still doing my washing or the career is off!' I burst into laughter, not just because me winning any awards was preposterous but because he was swinging his arms around ridiculously for dramatic effect.

'Hmm, and I suppose you're blaming my washing for this jumper being so snug,' I said, prodding his belly.

'What do you mean? I'm as fit as a butcher's dog. The doc said so. And anyway, if I lost weight and got any more sexy I'd have to beat them off with a stick – you couldn't take the competition, darling.'

This was classic Derek, always my biggest cheerleader, always giving me cheek. He said it was to 'keep my feet on the ground', but really it was because he knew without a doubt that we already had everything we cared about right there: our little family and our normal little life, with our wonderful friends around us.

Still, despite our usual banter and his eternal belief in me, I couldn't help but feel that, this new year, something rather magical was going on. Fresh opportunities, fresh hope, fresh outlooks. There was just a sense that, yes, it might be our year after all.

I was just home from my stint on *I'm A Celebrity ... Get Me Out of Here*, and I was relieved to have survived it without making a total fool of myself. I'd even managed to surprise myself by discovering some bravery I didn't know I had. The show is incredible, a juggernaut, requiring you to cross the globe, live with people you've never met before (and might have nothing in common with), and face some of your biggest fears. I'd had huge spiders crawling over my face, taken baths in smelly blood and guts, walked out on a wooden plank on the roof of a skyscraper 300 feet in the air. It had been terrifying, but also exhilarating.

Time in 'the jungle' affects everyone who takes part in the show in different ways. For me, it had brought my priorities into sharper focus. Being cut off from my family had heightened how much I valued them, and the seriously basic living had reminded me of just how lucky I was to have my comfortable life at home. Meeting new and fascinating people, and pushing myself to my physical limits, kind of revved me up and made me ready to take on new challenges, where once I would have shied away. And, thanks to the huge popularity of the show, new and interesting opportunities were coming my way in abundance.

By the first week of January I had been offered the pilot for a new quiz show for ITV (I'd always wanted to do a quiz show!), my own Saturday morning chat-show, which I was buzzing to get stuck into, and I was also working on new documentary ideas with other TV channels. I stood at the start of the new year feeling renewed, thinking I had survived the toughest experience of my life, faced my worst fears – separation, isolation, hunger, heights, snakes and all those creepy-crawlies – and thrived. Surely 2020 would be a breeze.

How wrong I was. That hadn't come anywhere close to the toughest experience of my life. My biggest challenge was just around the corner, and it was, for the most part, going to take place in my own home.

The first time I heard mention of coronavirus was in the newsroom at *Good Morning Britain*, an unfamiliar word in a foreign news feed. It felt distant, not just physically, but emotionally too. I'm not even sure we put those very early reports into our news bulletins. After all, why would an illness on the other side of the world have any resonance with someone waking up here in the UK? We have to make decisions all the time about what stories people will want to hear about, what news will have the most impact on their lives. At this point, without the knowledge of how it could spread, we wondered how it might affect our viewers. Why would they want to know about it? Back then there was far more focus on the impact of Brexit, on the decision that Harry and Meghan had taken to leave the Royal Family. It was much more obvious why those items might make people sit up and take notice.

It didn't seem like a headline but what we would call a 'middle bulletin' story. It wasn't a lead, which was reserved for events that directly impacted on our viewers' lives, or an 'and finally', a story to make you smile before heading out of the door. It was just sort of in the middle.

To me too it felt remote, not just because it was so far away, vague reports coming in from China, but also because news is my job. This belonged at work. It wasn't a story that would get any closer to me than reading the headlines. The notion was unimaginable that it would transform not just the world we lived in, but my family, my love, my friendships.

We continued to report on it as winter slowly became spring, from that first mention to the first case in the UK. Spring half-term came and went, and with it the so-called 'super-spreader' in Brighton, then the return of UK citizens from China's Hubei province, required to quarantine in Milton Keynes on arrival. We watched them while they disembarked as if it were a science-fiction show. It seemed that after their two weeks indoors the situation would be contained. We were told we were protected, so why should we doubt it?

Even when that turned out not to be true and the disease

began its creep into the UK, starting to dominate headlines as the number of cases grew, so many individual stories impossible to detail, I still never imagined it would affect me so directly. Or at least, if it did, that the preventive measures would hit us rather than ill health, and that even the ill health would have an impact only on the elderly or those with existing conditions.

Derek, ironically, *was* concerned. He read voraciously anyway, and now he was reading about this, not just the reports from here at home but, because he was so plugged into the business and political world internationally, reports from all over the globe too. He'd noticed clients were less keen to travel from abroad, and when I talked to him about plans for the school Easter holidays, he said simply, 'We'll be here, babe. No one will be flying anywhere for fun by then.'

By the beginning of February he had created a notice for the front door saying: *Anyone coming into the house, please wash your hands IMMEDIATELY. Do not touch anything before THOROUGHLY cleaning hands.*

It seemed brutal to me, even rude, that the first thing people saw coming to our front door was such a direct command, almost an insult to their cleanliness. And he was making the kids wash their hands so often that they were dry and raw, meaning I had to give them hand cream. The stark notice is still on the front door, the edges curling. No one has the heart to take it down and, sadly, the need for it to be there remains.

Derek's concerns sharpened my instinct to err on the safe

side. I made sure that I'd ordered a whole load of vitamins and supplements to boost the immune system and even some face masks, which were still in plentiful supply as we were not yet being told to wear them. I made sure I sent some to my parents as well as Derek's. I even got them some strange creams to go up the nose as I had read that inhalation might be how the virus infected us. I hadn't seen anything like it since using First Defence on long-haul flights, but it felt sensible to be belt and braces about things.

By early March, Covid was dominating *Good Morning Britain* but the bigger worries seemed to be peripheral things, like stockpiling. Social media was full of panicked images of supermarket shelves bare of flour, pasta and toilet rolls. We were being encouraged not to over-buy, but a part of me wondered if it was irresponsible not to prepare, and what else we could do. It seemed I wasn't alone: my eldest, Darcey, was developing quite a 'Dig for Britain' approach to the news and said to me, 'Mum, I think we should buy some seeds and bulbs. Maybe we need to grow our own fruit and veg this year.'

I'm a passionate gardener, but until that spring Darcey had never shown any interest. The idea of planting something, waiting and then seeing it peek up above the soil was way, way too slow for a teenager used to fifteen-second TikToks, but suddenly she was keen.

I couldn't say yes fast enough, and we headed off to the local garden centre the same afternoon. It was lovely weather, a perfect spring day before those slightly unnerving scorchers that came in April. We had our basket, we had a plan and we spent a joyful hour or two choosing. We picked raspberry and kiwi fruit plants, and radishes, carrots, cabbage and other seeds. For a while it felt as if we had the place to ourselves but a day or two later I noticed that everyone seemed to have had the same idea and they had run out of almost everything.

That afternoon, as we sat in their café, me with a cup of tea and Darcey having her cake, I really felt optimistic about what we could get out of this unusual era.

'This is going to be so much fun! Something to do if we go into full lockdown!' I told Darcey. 'We could even do a project about germination and show your teachers ...'

Darcey rolled her eyes. I had enjoyed seeing how far her enthusiasm might go, but it seemed I had reached her limit. Too far, Mum ... When we got home and were unloading the car, showing Derek our purchases as we brought them round to the garden, he had a good laugh at our antics.

Days later on 18 March came the news that the schools would be closing the following week. It was the first time I felt the sting of everyday life changing on a massive scale. Coronavirus had now well and truly seeped out from the safety of the headlines and into our lives. Despite that, it still seemed like an experience that might not be entirely negative. Of course I felt anxiety, just like everyone else, but also a sense that we were part of something bigger than ourselves, part of a collective effort. Something to experience as a family. Perhaps a bit more time at home together was something to be cherished. We might do some of the things we had always meant to do. We might come out of a fearful time a little closer, maybe even a little wiser. And certainly with a better garden.

That weekend Derek went to his office and got everything he needed to work at home. He is a psychologist; his business deals with leadership training, coaching and developing FTSE 100 companies. He was going to have to make the same shift to Zoom and Microsoft Teams that so many of us were, but it was relatively easy for him to move to home working as the news grew more serious with what seemed like every bulletin.

We decided to seize the moment and do the bits and pieces around the home that had been waiting for what seemed like for ever. Instead of leaving it on the back-burner, like we had done for years, we went out and bought a bunch of photo frames. We would hang our happy memories – the baby pictures, the wedding photos and all the rest – now, rather than waiting for the home improvements we had planned to be completed. Maybe we would make something of this. Maybe 2020 could still be our year after all.

Home schooling began on Monday, 23 March, and the full national lockdown followed the next day. As a family, we got ourselves set up and working in this strange new way without too much of a fuss. I was classed as a key worker, so I was still able to go into *Good Morning Britain* and to my Smooth Radio show at Global. But not without changes: safety precautions were starting to affect the way we worked. At Smooth, we started discussions about getting me a sort of home studio, 'just in case' the restrictions got tighter. We arranged to have the equipment set up that week, and to have rehearsals the following Monday. It seemed like sensible planning and there were positives: at least I could be around more to help Derek with the home schooling, we could spend proper time together, and we could be as safe as possible.

At ITV, furious planning was going on at senior level: how to keep on air while still keeping everyone safe. Shaking hands was out, even 'showbiz'-style air-kissing was deemed too close. We had fun thinking up different ways of saying hello. Remember the weird elbow-fencing memes? Or even the foot-crossing taps that left you looking like a clumsy Michael Flatley in *Riverdance*? Everyone seemed to mistime the supposed friendly greeting: you ended up kicking their ankle or having your shin clobbered. It seemed daft, contrived, not the serious life-saving measure it was supposed to be – and ended up as a bit of a joke.

In the *Good Morning Britain* newsroom we all had to separate and, even on set, sit apart from the other presenters. We teased each other about 'not getting too close', holding up tape measures to make sure we were exactly two metres apart. But I'm not sure any of us believed we were truly a danger to each other.

Much more concerning to me personally at that point was that I had something wrong with my eye. It was so sore and scratchy I couldn't put my contact lenses in, and meant I had to wear glasses on air, which normally I never do. Cue lots of teasing from Ben Shephard, my co-presenter, about trying to look more 'intelligent'. But one tweet from a concerned viewer struck an alarm bell.

'Is Kate's sore eye because she has conjunctivitis? Does she know that can be a symptom of coronavirus?'

Off camera, I asked Dr Hilary, who was usually only on the show for special medical features but by now was in the studio every day, addressing viewers' concerns about the virus. He said there had been some early medical reports that infections of the eye could be related to the virus but it was very unlikely and largely now dismissed. Certainly not a key symptom.

I was concerned enough, though, to feel I should get it looked at by an expert. Our GP surgery was swamped and only doing phone consultations, and we were being discouraged from troubling A & E, so I opted for the walk-in emergency clinic at Moorfields eye hospital and headed there as soon as I could. By then, Derek was also starting to feel a little under the weather. He had had a shoulder injury for a month or two and had been about to have steroid injections that week, but they were cancelled abruptly, along with so many other procedures considered non-urgent. His doctor had given him stronger painkillers and he presumed they were affecting him negatively so resolved to stop taking them. We didn't yet know otherwise.

At least I had good news: the problem with my eye was only a scratched cornea. The relief that I was not infected! I'd simply done something grim with my contact lens. When I got home that Thursday afternoon I still had the anaesthetic numbing solution the hospital had used in my eye, so everything seemed foggy and blurred. What I could see, though, was that Derek had loaded the dishwasher and cleaned the entire kitchen.

'My God, darling,' I said. 'You *must* be feeling out of sorts. This is only about the second time you've done that in our entire marriage. Who are you and what have you done with Derek Draper?'

At first I was delighted that he was turning into such a homebody, but then I realized it was because he had got as much of the house in order as possible so that he could go to bed the minute I got back. Normally he took care of the kids on a Thursday evening, leaving me to prepare for my *Good Morning Britain* early shift the next day. But this time he looked desperate. Looking after two children new to home schooling while I was out all day had clearly left him wiped out, and I took pity on him. But none of us was worried. If anything, we were relieved that my eye had turned out not to be anything serious.

That evening was the first national Clap for Carers, which we were supporting at Global Radio and I had been promoting all week on Smooth. It seemed like such a wonderful idea, offering thanks to the caregivers, who were under so much pressure. It was already dark at 8 p.m. and as the kids and I got ready to go out I couldn't help wondering if anyone would actually do it. Did anyone really know what was going on and feel the urge to get involved, show such a bold spirit of community? But before we could even open the door we heard the roar, ripples of clapping and cheering as neighbours in every house had come out and were standing on the steps waving and whooping. It was such a wonderful and emotional moment of love and togetherness that I found my eyes filling with tears. The kids were moved too, screaming, 'We have to get Dad up. He's got to see this!' Who knew back then it was the start of so many Claps for Carers, and how could I have known just how much they would carry me through so many tough Thursday nights over the next ten weeks? Back then, it just felt like a one-off special event that we were so pleased to have been part of.

The headlines the next morning, Friday 27 March, were filled with Covid-19 stories: doctors were being asked to sleep on site in hospitals and nurses were being transferred to the capital. 'London faces a tsunami of Covid-19 patients within days' was our headline on *Good Morning Britain*, which I knew to be true – but as I delivered it on air it felt almost surreal, like I was playing the part of a newscaster in a Hollywood movie. I felt sick: this was real, happening right now all around us. We talked about Clap for Carers, the success of which had left us all still moved. After the headlines, I put up with Ben's teasing about my glasses, explaining that I wasn't trying to look clever by wearing specs but that I had been to the hospital, partly thanks to the concern from our viewers.

'They took my temperature and checked my chest, and I'm perfect!' I added. And we got on with the rest of the show.

Unaware of what was to come.

Meanwhile, at home, Derek had woken up with a splitting headache and pain in his sinuses. Later that morning he rang to say he wondered if it was sinusitis so I called our GP to discuss it. She asked if he had a temperature or a cough.

And when I said no cough and no temperature, she sounded brighter, 'Right, sinusitis, then,' and immediately prescribed antibiotics without question. It felt as if doctors were doing whatever they could to keep people with anything other than Covid safe and at home, even if it meant doling out drugs like sweeties.

When I came off air at Smooth Radio a few hours later I ran a couple of errands, including picking up Derek's prescription, and made my way home. At 3 p.m. I received a text from him:

Are you near? Please be near? I feel terrible.

Derek is absolutely not someone who gets man-flu twice a year and behaves as if the world is ending. It's just not his style. He rarely gets ill, and even when he does, yes, of course he demands lots of attention, but always with his tongue in his cheek. There was something unsettling about this curt text. Then minutes later another:

Are you near? Please be near?

This was not like him at all. He sounded desperate. I got home as quickly as I could and was relieved when I walked in to see him out of bed and watching Billy playing with his Lego. He did look unwell, though, and as I found him something to take the first antibiotics with I couldn't help but ask, 'Derek, we aren't missing the obvious here, are we? This isn't Covid, is it?'

21

Saying it out loud, I was worried I'd freak him out, but he had obviously been thinking the same.

'I had that fear in the night too. I've been taking my temperature all day and it's definitely not up. And I don't have a cough either.'

Back then, no one knew about the array of other symptoms to look out for and the advice was very clear: if you don't have a continuous cough or a rise in temperature, it's not Covid. All the same, as I sent him back to bed for a rest, I couldn't help taking his temperature again, just to be sure. He was right.

Over the weekend Derek seemed to rally, and we ended up having a lovely family time. We worked on the garden, we sorted some of the photo frames, and we really, properly enjoyed each other's company. As we went to bed on Sunday night he said he felt much better and that the antibiotics seemed to be working.

But things were very different when I returned from work on Monday: Derek looked unmistakably terrible. Pale, clammy, exhausted. And dispirited.

'I think you're really ill,' I told him. 'I'm getting scared now but I'm not sure what to do because you haven't even got a hint of a temperature.'

The headlines were so clear: a sky-high temperature and a continuous cough were the only symptoms we should bother a doctor with. Anything else might mean clogging up the system. But he looked so profoundly ill that my every instinct was saying I shouldn't ignore this.

I paced up and down the bedroom for a bit while he lay on our bed saying very little. I tried ringing 111, I tried the GP, and I even thought about ringing the emergency services. But with no proper symptoms? Was I really that person? After all, that was exactly what I had been encouraging people on air *not* to do. Instead, I did what every single person who has ever worked in breakfast TV does at some point: I called Dr Hilary Jones.

'I don't know what to do because I don't want to waste the time of the emergency services, but he's so ill. I'm just not sure when to worry if it's Covid.'

The first thing Dr Hilary did was to ask if I was OK, and I said I was fine, apart from my eye driving me mad. Then he asked me to put Derek on the phone. I could hear him asking some basic questions. Then he asked Derek to do a couple of breathing tests, holding his breath for certain amounts of time and so on. After a minute or two Derek handed the phone back, apparently unworried.

But I will never forget what I heard next.

'You need to call an ambulance. Now,' said Dr Hilary.

'Really?'

'Yes.' He was completely serious, which I was not prepared for. 'It's worrying. His breathing really is not right.'

I had been asking Derek if his chest felt tight as he wasn't coughing, and now I asked him if he felt he couldn't breathe.

'No, my head is just killing me, and my sinuses. But it doesn't feel like my chest at all.'

But Dr Hilary had spoken, so I called an ambulance. Even as I was calling it, I could hear myself having said on air only hours earlier that you shouldn't call unless you had those very specific symptoms. I was thinking it was going to be so embarrassing, that the crew would arrive, take one look at someone off the telly and go, 'Oh for God's sake …' But Dr Hilary had left no room for doubt, and now they were on their way.

I went downstairs and tidied the house, moving my work bag out of the hallway, running up to move anything that had been left on the stairs, just making things presentable in that very British way. The ambulance crew might judge me for being neurotic enough to call them, but at least they wouldn't be able to judge my messy house.

When they arrived, a crew of two women, the first thing they asked, while still standing back on the pavement, was, 'Is he breathing?' I said yes. 'OK, give us a minute.' They went to the vehicle and put their PPE on. We were still in that slightly muddled stage when we were told that masks for ordinary people would do more harm than good as they encouraged you to touch your face, but there was no hesitation as they donned plastic aprons, paper masks and gloves, not the full suits we all saw later in intensive-care units.

Ambulance crews are trained to be calm, but I remember noting how measured and reassuring those two were. They came upstairs to Derek, put a mask on him too, took a pin-prick of blood, and said within seconds that his oxygen levels were very, very low, and that he had to come to hospital immediately. I felt an icy panic creep over me, wondering if the children could hear any of this from downstairs, how I was going to tell them. But I knew I had to hold things together. Derek was flustered, not about being sick but that he didn't have a bag packed. He had never been to hospital before. The only time he had ever been on a ward as anything like a patient was when the children were born and that was completely different – exciting. Good news, not an unexpected plunging into international events.

I told him not to worry and started to put together some bits, but after a minute or two I realized that the ambulance crew had a very definite air of urgency about them.

'No, don't worry about that,' they said. And to me: 'You're not going to be able to come.'

The mood in the room changed.

Derek and I spend very little time apart. It felt as if we had only just been reunited after my time in the jungle, and now we were being told that I wasn't allowed to accompany him to what was arguably one of the most frightening moments he had ever faced. I just wanted to hold his hand and reassure him. But what could we do? Neither of us disputed the safety measures the hospitals were putting in place. But fear was creeping into our home, faster and faster with every passing minute.

For a moment, things seemed a little lighter at the sight of these two women trying to help Derek, who is six foot two and was determined to walk down the stairs towards the ambulance. But by the time we reached the hallway we saw that Darcey and Billy had heard the kerfuffle and appeared at the bottom of the stairs, looking really scared. How strange that such a short time ago I had been tidying there, as if that might be the biggest problem the visit presented.

'Don't worry, guys. They're just going to help me get better, to check me over …' he explained. But that didn't reassure any of us.

Moments later, Derek was in the back of the ambulance with a mask on, receiving oxygen. When Darcey and Billy followed us out, he began trying to point, the tubes for the oxygen twisting around his arm as he attempted to usher them back into the house. I encouraged them to stay inside while we got things sorted, that I would be back in a minute.

'Can I follow you to the hospital in the car?' I asked Derek.

'No, don't do that,' he said, lifting the oxygen mask from his face, his tone even sterner than his expression. I realized he was worried about the children being left home alone after seeing what they just had. He wanted things to be as undisturbed as possible for them. He knew they needed me, and he was right. But my heart was hammering at the thought of saying goodbye to him, seeing him disappear down the road, not knowing what he would face when he got to the hospital.

I felt my blood run cold as one of the paramedics went to close the ambulance doors, finally obscuring my view of him. I had a strange, all-consuming feeling rush through me, and Derek must have picked up on it.

'Kate,' he said, lifting the mask from his mouth again. 'This is *not* the last time you will see me. It isn't.'

But I knew that he would never have said that if at least a small part of him hadn't been wondering if it was. He was absolutely terrified and it showed on his face. I tried to keep my voice steady. 'I know it's not. Of course it's not!' I replied. 'I love you.'

It felt as if it was happening to someone else, not us. I was part of the story I had been reporting on for so long in the worst way possible. As I watched the ambulance back discreetly down the road before turning on the blues and twos and speeding away, sirens blaring, I felt like an actor playing me. Externally I wasn't freaking out. Maybe the decades of coping with live breaking news stories on TV had taught me how to keep a steady composure, an air of calm, even when all hell was breaking loose. I knew that the hospitals were nearly overwhelmed. I had read those headlines about the tsunami of patients only hours before. I was sure that he was going to the right place for him, but felt uncomfortable that I couldn't be there with him, be an advocate for him. So as I crossed the threshold back into the family home I was showing nothing, but inside I was queasy with the knowledge that all was far from well.

'Right, guys,' I said to the kids, trying to keep my voice as breezy as possible. 'Dad is definitely going to be staying in overnight so the doctors can help him get better. Let's get ourselves sorted with some food. I'm going to be busy for a bit making some phone calls.'

'Staying overnight?' said Billy, his eyes widening with worry.

'Yes, just to do proper checks. It's late anyway now, so he'll want to get some sleep.'

I tried to sound reassuring.

'Can we watch TV in your bed? Snuggle down together?'

asked Darcey. She was trying her luck as she knew this was a treat. I must have said yes too quickly because this time it was her turn to widen her eyes and I knew she was thinking, This must be serious. Mum's already relaxing the rules.

But before I had a chance to say more my phone rang.

It was my editor from *Good Morning Britain*, Neil Thompson, who, by chance, had called to talk about changes to my shift pattern.

'My God!' I said. 'Derek's just been taken away in an ambulance. They think he might even have Covid.'

Neil's tone changed in a heartbeat. 'Right. Your priority now is not us, or rosters, or any of that. You need to go through to the next room and see your children. You need to show them that they're safe. They need you.'

'I am, I am …' I protested.

'No, Kate, I mean it. Your priority isn't even Derek right now. He's getting the care he needs. It's those children.'

'Yes, yes, you're right …'

I hung up, then set about making snacks and tidying up. Later we cuddled down in bed together, all three of us. Derek texted to say he had arrived and was waiting to be seen. He sounded upbeat, and said he wouldn't be able to call but was going to try to get some sleep. I was to give the kids a big kiss and get some sleep myself. Eventually the kids did fall asleep, but there was no chance for me. I slipped out of the bed and started to make my calls, including the grim one to Derek's parents, who were obviously terrified. But there seemed nothing else we could do until we knew more.

The next day Derek rang to say he was still in A & E, just waiting to be cleared for a bed. Neither of us knew that it would be intensive care. He told me that it was actually a relief to be there, to feel that the doctors were on the case.

'It's so loud here, though,' he said. 'It's total chaos. Could you bring my noise-cancelling headphones?'

I didn't like the sound of things in the hospital, but the good news was that I was allowed to bring him the headphones, if I also brought the device that he used for his sleep apnoea: it had an attached mask to breathe through. This worried me as it raised the suggestion that they might not have enough masks or breathing apparatus at the hospital, but I was just so pleased to be able to see him that I shoved that thought to the back of my mind.

I got the kids to write him notes saying they missed him, telling him what they had had for tea, and so on. Anything to let him know we were thinking of him and that we were all OK. Then I grabbed the headphones and leapt into the car as fast as I could. I arrived at the hospital eagerly clutching the things Derek had asked for, but I hadn't even reached the door before someone came out in full PPE, asked me to put his belongings into a plastic bag and said I would not be allowed to come any closer, let alone into the building.

'Please can I come in?' I begged. But the answer was unmoving: you can't.

When I got home, Derek had texted some photographs to Darcey and Billy, showing them who his doctors were. It felt reassuring. But from those messages onwards, we weren't so much constantly in touch as constantly *trying* to be in touch. Derek's messages were increasingly sporadic and confusing. I didn't know then that he wasn't starting to get better. He was getting worse; his breathing was harder and his lungs were ceasing to function properly. And he was trying to keep the worst of it from us:

22.27 Still can't phone, but all good. X-ray was positive. Thank you for your lovely notes. Love you all, won't be able to reply.

I texted back:

Love you very much. Slightly hysterical at the thought of you there on your own, but just know we're all thinking of you. Darcey has made a den in her bedroom and has Bill up there with her, mothering him. She won't admit she is worried. Typical Darcey, she is coping in her own way.

Reassuring to be here. Still can't come off the breathing machine for one minute so not allowed and can't talk. Please bring wax earphones, the soundproof headphones aren't enough it's just so noisy. They are on top of the new cupboard with my Mexican skulls. I will text you the ward name to bring them to when I get it. Love you all – say hello to Bill and Darcey. They say I am making an improvement.

A few hours later the hospital called: they were still trying to find space on a ward for Derek, possibly an intensive-care unit. This didn't sound like the improvement Derek had mentioned, but the person who informed me was just passing on a message and was unable to answer any questions. I was starting to learn that communication was almost impossible. Things were not functioning normally. You couldn't speak to a doctor or nurse as they were just too busy to pick up the phone, and if the phone was picked up, it would be in a completely different part of the hospital from the extension I had rung. On the occasions I got through to someone, the background noise was so extreme it was hard to hear what they were saying. And sometimes all they could do was say 'We can't talk, we can't talk' and hang up. The last thing I wanted to do was to distract them from dealing with the people needing help.

Eventually a consultant called and briefed me. I immediately texted Derek:

> I've spoken to your consultant. He says you're improving. Bill and Darcey send love.

He replied with a stream of kisses.

> I know you can't speak but I just want to know how the night went. They won't update me until 2 p.m. at the earliest and anyway I can't get through to the hospital. If there is any way you can get a nurse to call me with your oxygen breathing levels please do.

He texted back four hours later.

> I can't do anything. But I think you should ask Dave and
> Tiffy [who are my cousins] to drive down and live with
> the kids and you should call an ambulance. I'm really
> worried for you.

Why on earth was he worried about me? I replied quickly:

> Why are you worried about me? I'm fine. It's all good
> here.

> OK. Love you.

Then it dawned on me that he must have thought I was
getting sick, that I would be as ill as him before too long,
and the kids would be in danger.

Later on I did end up with Covid (though, mercifully,
never as badly as Derek), but at this point me being sick was
the furthest thing from my mind. All of my attention was
focused on Derek and the kids and, of course, we three had
been in self-isolation from the moment he was taken into
hospital to ensure there was no risk of us passing anything
on to anyone else. I had so much adrenalin coursing through
my veins and was getting so little sleep that I was barely in
touch with anything going on in my own body.

My friend Piers Morgan thinks that's what got me through
those first days. 'You are a journalist, Kate. Use those skills
and the adrenalin. Treat this as the biggest story of your life

… Getting the best for Derek is your goal and use that focus to hold yourself together.' And it helped. Tapping into my professional problem-solving and fact-finding skills helped me to manage the devastating pain and worry, and prevented me from folding into a total emotional mess. I called anyone who had medical contacts, and within a day or two I had spoken to everyone I knew who knew a doctor. I just had to monitor things, I told myself, and then I might be able to work out the best way to help. There was no point in letting the raw terror take over: it would only get in the way. I was determined to find the facts I needed to help Derek get well again. At the very least I could feel I was doing something positive – I felt so helpless being cut off from him, not even able to get through on the phone.

Later the consultant called and confirmed Derek had tested positive for Covid. It had been obvious from the start that they were treating him as a Covid case but without any of the usual symptoms. A part of me had clung to a fragment of hope it might be something else, something less devastating, something curable. But just as I was taking that in, he delivered worse news. Derek's breathing capacity had gone down significantly and they were now considering putting him into an induced coma. I tried to stay calm, and explained that I had a selection of things he had asked for and could I bring them to the hospital. Again, they said they wouldn't let me in, but I could drop items off.

I scrambled together snacks for the kids to distract them, warned them to keep the phone next to them and not to answer the door to anyone until I got back. And then I rushed off. At the hospital I couldn't even get into the car park: cordons were zigzagging across the entrance. I got as close as I could, abandoning the car on the edge of the grounds, and ran to A & E Reception.

A nurse came out to meet me and I was astounded when she said I could come in. My heart leapt with excitement because I was going to get a chance to see Derek – then plunged as I saw from the seriousness of the nurse's expression that this change of heart, this bending of the rules, could not mean good news. Oh God, was this *it?* Were they letting me in because he was slipping away? Was he actually going to die? It reminded me of the combined sense of urgency and foreboding that I used to feel in the playground when the kids were younger and one would fall over: part of me would be desperate, rushing over, heart full of love, to help come what may, while another was feeling the first queasy slosh of adrenalin as I realized I had no idea what I would see when I lifted my child's face from the bottom of the climbing frame. Would teeth be missing, their nose broken? Would there be blood everywhere?

I had to get into full PPE kit outside the hospital. I was wearing jeans and a jumper when I arrived, and now I was given a pair of plastic trousers to slip on over the top and a smock-shaped plastic gown that tied at the back (like the sort of thing you're given at the hairdresser's), which I was told to tuck into the trousers. I put plastic gloves over my hands, a second pair over the first, which they sealed with an elastic band over the gown's plastic sleeves. I had already been asked to tie my hair back, and now I had to put on a shower-cap-style hat and a mask. Once I had the full kit on, I was allowed to head into the hospital.

I followed the nurse straight through A & E and past the desk where you would normally check in. It was a warm day, but I felt the temperature rising – whether from within me and my now-racing heart or the heat in the hospital I'll never know.

As my anxiety mounted and the noise around me grew, I could focus only on that nurse's face. Everything else seemed to shift out of focus, into a blur, as if my eyes could take nothing more in. My heart continued to swing almost violently between desperation to see Derek and blind panic.

Then we reached the Red Area. What a horrible expression, I thought. I just want to go to the area where everything is all right. The lilac area, where everything is getting better. Or the beige area where everything is boringly undramatic. The noise grew as we went through pair after pair of swing doors.

We covered our already double-gloved hands with antibacterial gel, and finally turned left, before reaching Derek, face down on a stretcher, still waiting for a bed.

I gasped as I saw him and was glad the angle at which he was lying meant he couldn't see my reaction. He looked horrific. His skin was waxy and so pale he almost looked an icy blue. He was shivering and drenched in sweat, although they were still saying he didn't have a temperature. It was just pouring off him. It was obvious that he had no oxygen in his blood, that he really was incredibly sick.

I had hoped he might be on a ward, safe and getting

treatment, but I realized he had effectively been in A & E all of this time. It was hard for us to see each other because he was lying on his front. I asked if I could touch him, which was met with a regretful but firm no from the nurse who had led me in. I bent down so he could see me and kept telling him that we loved him.

I don't know how much he could hear or even understand. He seemed almost delirious, muttering again and again that he loved me. Then, amid the declarations of love, he started to talk about a funeral. It took me a minute to realize that he was talking about his own.

'I want you at the funeral,' he said, his voice very weak. 'But I'm not sure about the children.'

Even saying that made him choke. He was gasping for breath, as if he had run a sprint in a smoke-filled room or was drowning in front of me. The sound was unbearably frightening. My blood felt cold, but I knew it was up to me to get him through the next few moments.

'Don't be daft. Stop talking about funerals, no one is going to a funeral. You've got to fight this,' I told him. 'You *have* to get through it. You're so determined, you can do it. You can get through it. I'm in touch with the doctors, and they say you're doing better. Stick with it …' I kept repeating myself, almost like a mantra.

I looked around me and asked what was going on, what they were going to do, and I was told they were trying their very best to get his oxygen levels up, and to find a ward with a ventilator. I couldn't leave him like that. 'Look, I need to speak to somebody.'

But I was told I had to leave. They promised that someone would call me soon, but that I absolutely had to go. I told Derek I had to leave. In between breaths, he managed to tell me to send love to Billy and Darcey, and to beg me not to tell them what I had seen.

Moments later, the double doors were swinging behind me, and I was back out of the Red Area, and into my new future.

Chapter 2

It's Not Fair

___

When I got back to my car it was several minutes before I could even consider driving. I just sat there, feeling empty, staring into space, reliving the last few minutes I'd spent with Derek. What if they were our last few minutes ever? I felt cold and nauseous.

Oh God, I thought, I just want to go back in and say everything again but better – and now I can't.

Then, in a flash, I snapped back into the present. The kids! I had to get home to them, and then, with a second wave of nausea, what on earth was I going to tell them?

I drove home with my mind running potential explanations over and over again. I didn't want to lie to them or give them false promises but also didn't want to show them how scared I was. They were used to me being the calm one, the one to offer a comforting hug and who would always reassure them with a 'Don't worry, we can sort this.' But 'this' I couldn't sort. How could I, when even the doctors weren't confident they could? I had to steady myself and manage my fears to a degree where I could help the kids feel safe and secure enough to face whatever was to come.

As I pulled up outside our house, Dr Hilary called my mobile. 'Just checking in to see how things are going,' he said, in his soothing way. I hadn't spoken to him since he had advised me to call the ambulance – just days ago, but it felt like weeks. He had no idea the situation had moved so fast. I explained everything to him, surprising myself with how much medical detail about blood-oxygen levels and breathing percentages I had taken in. He was his usual calm, comforting self, but his tone was serious as he reassured me that Derek was in the right place, that he could at last rest when he made it to a ward, that the NHS was going to take care of him. And that, because of his young age and lack of underlying conditions, he stood a good chance. I wanted to believe him. I wanted to so, so much.

Instead, I sat in the car for another minute, gathering my thoughts before heading in to Darcey and Billy. The one thing Derek had always said about children was that their fertile imaginations would be worse than any truth. If you tell children a lie, they will find out, and then they're faced with not just the thing you were trying to protect them from but also the shock of being lied to by someone close to them. And that destroys trust, which shakes them even further.

They had been to hospital on various occasions. Darcey had broken her arm when she was younger and Billy had been to A & E for twisted ankles and the usual scrapes and bruises. Crucially, however, they had only ever experienced doctors making them better: you go to hospital to get mended. They give you what you need, you're grateful, and you move on. So they weren't scared of the hospital *per se*. To them it was not somewhere a person never returns from. And I wanted to keep it that way.

I headed in and told them Dad had got the notes they'd written him, and that he loved them. I explained that he was feeling really bad, but he was doing well, and the doctors were doing everything they could to help. I never said to them, 'Don't worry, Daddy's not going to die.' That was a conscious decision. I didn't want them to think I even considered that a possibility, but I also didn't want to make a promise to them that I could not guarantee. And I couldn't help but notice that they didn't ask that question either, or at least not for a very long time after this. Perhaps they knew that if they asked they wouldn't like the answer, or perhaps they just never dared put it into words at this point. I also suspect that they wouldn't believe he could even be that sick. To be honest, I could hardly believe it myself. It was all so surreal ... and yet so real.

I quickly threw myself into normal 'mum stuff' to distract them: picking up discarded shoes and hoodies from the floor and lightly ticking them off for the mess, then getting tea on. Darcey, always practical, asked if she could help me cook – I knew this was her way of trying to feel close to me as well as help. We started getting the pans out, but before long I was back on the phone, updating Derek's parents and his sisters. While I paced, muttering into the phone as discreetly as I could, Darcey took charge in the kitchen, making us all a stir-fry. As we sat at the table, talking about YouTubers and music – anything but the news and the world outside – a passerby would never have suspected that this family was anything other than perfectly happy.

A couple of hours later, Billy asked again if he could watch TV in my bed, and this time Darcey wanted to join him. To my surprise, they asked if they could watch *Father Brown*. It's hardly the kind of show that would typically capture their imagination – a cosy daytime TV series about a Catholic priest solving crimes in 1950s England – but I think they associated it with me being calm and happy. For years it would air in the early afternoon around the time I came home from work at *Good Morning Britain* and Smooth, when I would try to get an hour or so's sleep before heading to do primary-school pick-up for Billy and Darcey. I would only ever manage to watch ten minutes or so before I fell asleep, so it would take me at least a week to watch an entire episode – I had long joked about the show's incredible soothing powers. And now it seemed that they fancied some of the comfort viewing for themselves.

Eight series were available, so we decided to start from the very beginning and watch it together as a sort of lockdown project. If everyone else was embarking on making sourdough or reading the complete George Smiley novels, why couldn't *we* watch all of *Father Brown* – surely life would be back to normal by the time we'd finished all eight series. And so began a tradition of the three of us curling up in bed to watch Mark Williams fighting crime in the gentlest way possible. In time, what would often follow was me creeping out of the room once they were asleep, and starting on another round of calls. To family, to experts, to friends, to the hospital once again … just in case this time I got through.

That night, just as I left the bedroom, I finally received the call I needed: an actual expert. By this stage, I'd realized that having Dr Hilary's direct line – although brilliant – wasn't enough. I needed someone who was dealing directly with Derek, in the thick of it, seeing things unfold moment by moment, not least because the situation was changing so fast, and the doctors' understanding of the virus with it.

It was midnight when a consultant from the hospital rang, Dr M, explaining he was one of those in charge of intensive care and had been working on Derek.

'Great to make contact with you,' I said, bracing myself for some complicated medical terms.

Instead, he simply said, 'Listen, he's really very sick. But so are so many others. We have some ventilators but we need more. We're trying really hard to source them but so is every other hospital, and we're trying to get him a bed in ICU.'

I didn't reply, slightly taken aback by a combination of this straight talking and how very posh the voice delivering it was. Then he continued, 'There's no doubt about it, your husband's on a sticky wicket … but we're going to get through it.'

I was sure he was moments from a 'Bally-ho!' It was all very Boris Johnson.

He meant well but I wanted facts before chummy reassurance. My only reply was, 'Fine, but what about these ventilators? What's going on?'

Which I suppose made him realize he could share with me the truth: I wasn't going to react hysterically.

There was a pause, then, in a softer voice, 'It's like the Somme … In this hospital, this week, it's like the bloody Somme. All around us people are just dying as we fight to save them. I am just coming off a thirty-six-hour shift, and I have never in my career known anything like this.'

Being told the truth like that, shocking though it was, strangely helped. I felt included, that we were allies not adversaries, that I wasn't someone to be palmed off and dismissed.

'I get it. What can I do to help?'

'I'll let you know. But things are very tough. We aren't just running out of ventilators, we are also running very low on oxygen to put through them. As you can imagine, the need for both has gone from virtually nought to ninety and the demand is just too high.'

He also explained that he would have liked to do all sorts of scans on Derek too, but it simply hadn't been possible. Derek had been complaining of a severe headache and in other circumstances they might have done an MRI, but that was impossible. The practical challenge of sanitizing the machines after a suspected Covid patient could take up to fourteen hours. They couldn't scan each and every case to check every symptom, especially as medical attention was focused on the lungs.

This was the reality of life behind the Covid headlines that only days ago I had been announcing on TV: the pressure on the NHS, overworked staff who were in danger of being overwhelmed, equipment and bed shortages. But hearing the reality and understanding the detail was terrifying. Derek was now living the headlines, and so was I.

Being told the truth focused my mind. I thanked Dr M – he was clearly very experienced, an expert at his job and doing his very best. There was still something unnerving about having spoken to the best of the best, though: if he couldn't be certain he could help Derek, *who could*? Well, I was going to try. At least that would make me feel I was doing something practical rather than just being helpless, cut off, waiting for news.

I spent the rest of the night on the phone with a friend who is a nurse in Kent, who could access the NHS's system. We spent hour after hour trying to see where in the country might have ventilators and how we could get them to Derek's hospital. She eventually found there were some in Bromley, not far from London. Maybe I could suggest that to the doctors in the morning: it might support their efforts for everyone they were trying to save as well as Derek.

Doing something, anything, relaxed me enough to nod off to sleep on the sofa. Suddenly the phone rang. I woke up and scrambled to answer.

From the first 'Hello, is that Mrs Draper?' I could tell something had changed, and not for the better. It was a nutritionist at the hospital who had been drafted in to help with the surge in family enquiries. She said she couldn't answer specific questions but wanted to let me know that Derek was struggling to breathe, even with support, and they were still considering putting him into an induced coma 'to give his lungs a rest', as she put it. They were waiting for a ventilator to become free. I told her that I had found some in another borough and she said she would pass it on. But I could tell she was under pressure to move on to her next call, to update another worried relative desperate for news. She reassured me that someone would be in touch to let me know which ward Derek would be on, and if I hadn't heard I should call back.

The rest of the day was a sort of endless torture. Trying to get hold of the hospital … and failing. Spending ninety minutes dialling the hospital … only to have someone pick up and say, 'We can't speak to you,' then hang up before you could draw breath to answer.

I kept trying, but even on the few occasions someone would answer, it was almost impossible to hear anything they were saying. Normally if you call a hospital it's quiet in the background, isn't it? You can maybe hear the odd ping of a machine, or someone quietly chatting nearby. But this was a deafening roar. It reminded me of the times I had called someone at a football match or a gig. A huge white noise of people shouting instructions and screaming at each other. It sounded like chaos and panic.

'It's so frustrating!' I kept muttering to myself. But it was more than that: it was frightening. It was terrifying.

I'll just go. I'll just get in the car and go to the hospital. I'll just barge my way in even if they don't want to let me in.

These were the thoughts racing through my mind, as I kept pacing the house, dialling the hospital until I was sick of the sight of the white of my thumb, pressing redial again and again.

But I knew I couldn't do it. They had told me firmly I wouldn't be let in under any circumstances: there was a rope cordon around the entrances to stop anyone even getting near. And if they were facing a situation as dire as running out of oxygen, of course they didn't have time to explain things to me. I would only make things worse.

Then I finally got through only for a nurse to say, 'I'm afraid I can't speak to you about this patient ... I ... don't know where he is ... his name isn't here any more ...'

'What? *What?*' I asked. This change in tone could mean the worst news of all.

'I'm not allowed—'

'Has he DIED?'

No reply.

'Don't hang up on me! Don't hang up until you know!' I was desperate.

I could hear the panic mounting in the nurse's voice, the shuffling of paper, the thud of a handset being put down as the line was still open. Muttering. My heart beating, surely audible during this silence. I felt for the nurse almost as much as myself during that never-ending pause. I knew staff had been drafted in from everywhere, I had seen the mayhem on the ward. I had heard the commotion on my previous calls. I waited.

'I've got to go, I have to help someone …' was all she said before the line went dead.

For the next few hours I tried to call other numbers I had. Anyone, anywhere in the hospital. Sweat flushed my entire body. Words I would use to tell the children the feared bad news flooded my mind. I felt faint but couldn't do anything but keep trying. I *had* to know.

Eventually, I got through and was told that they had located Mr Draper, and that he was being looked after. It seemed he had a similar name to someone who had died, and the nurse knew she couldn't be the one to tell me, especially as she wasn't sure. With all the patients lying down with oxygen masks on it must be impossible to tell them apart, especially as there were so many people running around – did anyone know who was who?

I put the phone down, went into the bathroom, locked the door behind me, and shouted, 'I'll just be a minute, guys!' Leaning with my back against the door, I felt almost delirious with relief. But then the sheer horror that someone, not that far away, was being delivered the opposite news.

In that moment I saw so clearly, and muttered to myself, 'This is a living hell. And there are thousands if not more across the whole country stuck in it, like me.'

I splashed some cold water on my face, looked in the mirror and took a deep breath, then headed back out to take control of the only thing I could: being a mother.

The next text I sent to Derek was a picture of Billy holding a Legends character, a plastic figure Derek had ordered for him while they were together only a few days earlier.

> It's arrived, Bill says thank you! Hope you're feeling
> better.

It was only days but it felt like weeks since Derek had been
at home. He replied pretty quickly.

> Hi Bill, that looks cool. Feeling a bit better, but really
> missing you, Dada and Mum.

Such relief.

I smiled at the sight of Darcey's family nickname, as
coined by baby Billy, coming up on my phone. A shard of
normality, of life between the four of us, amid the chaos and
fear. I replied quickly:

> Oh my God we're all crying. Well not Dada, who never
> thought you would die anyway.

I knew that by mentioning Darcey's confidence I was imply-
ing that she *had* been worried Derek would die – and I was
suddenly worried Derek would pick up on that too. But before
I could send another text reassuring him, Derek had replied.

> I miss you all so much. Can't wait to see you. Right,
> mask back on now.

Then there was nothing until 7 p.m., by which point I had
been informed that he was on a ward – and that by now
most of the wards in the hospital were dealing with Covid

cases. We received a text complete with a photograph of Derek in bed, a smiling doctor by his side. It was addressed to Darcey and Billy:

> Greetings. It is still hard work but Dr Sarah says I am improving, bit by bit. I love you both so much. I get to take this mask off for ten seconds an hour, and my food is that little lilac cube. It goes into the mask and up to my nostrils and straight to my stomach. Anyway, love you all, everyone going to bed here.

My reply was swift.

> Jesus, love you so much. Please keep fighting, nothing works without you.

Reading this back today, I can see that my façade was cracking. I was really feeling the strain of keeping everything going at home, as well as keeping up the pressure at the hospital, and was worried I was about to start unravelling. And then I read his next text:

> OK, not for the kids. I've been playing down how really awful it is. It is second after second of being locked in a mask thinking every second you're going to die. I think they now may want to put me to sleep.

He was referring to the managed coma the doctors had already mentioned to me.

I'm terrified, but I can't take one more fucking hour of this. I'm sure you'll get to talk to the doctor. I want him to call you.

Oh my god, darling. I love you so much. Please, please stay strong. Please get the doctor to call.

And then three hours went by with nothing. By now it was lunchtime on Friday. I typed:

Please, please, please get someone to call me.

All I had been doing between those two messages was texting and trying to call. And absolutely no one was picking up. The kids were being so good, it hurts my heart to think of it now. I was in a frenzy on my phone, just saying yes to Fortnite for six hours in a row. *No problem. Don't worry about home school!*

Finally he replied:

They don't pick up full stop. If it is going to happen, you will be consulted. But it's looking less likely now. The phone is constantly ringing and no one has got time to pick up. People have died around me.

I felt sick.

I just want to check your blood oxygen levels.

I had, as you may have realized by now, become obsessed by getting his blood-oxygen levels and any medical detail I could. Because contact was so haphazard and you never spoke to the same person twice, when I did get through it was something concrete I could ask staff to check. A way of measuring his progress up or down. On the few times I ever managed to get hold of anyone in the week since Derek had been admitted, they didn't know who I was or what I knew. They would start off with 'Yes, yes, don't worry, he's doing well,' and then if I asked more they would try to explain the whole story from the start, which I knew no one had time for. So I decided if I could get at least one figure out of them, I could compare with the previous time. They could quickly tell me, 'It's up to 70 per cent now,' or 'I'm sorry but it's down to 40 per cent at the moment' and I would fit that into a bigger picture.

Eventually, as the months were to go by, I started to understand how to ask for liver-function indicator levels, kidney levels, and the rest, to be in with a chance of under-standing more. I have box files' worth of notes now, as my knowledge has grown. But I had learnt in the worst possible way that the people in the ward that first week could barely tell Derek apart from any of their other patients, so I didn't want to get lost in all that they were enduring, or indeed contribute to it. I just wanted the data, and I worked out that if I could get anyone to give me those blood-oxygen levels, I could at least monitor the very base of the problem.

Derek had clearly understood this, and was trying to keep me calm:

Discussions are still going on here. They have stepped
up their game. Thank you for talking to Dr M because
he came in person.

So he knew that I was virtually stalking this poor consultant who was working night and day in the hardest of
conditions. It probably would have made him laugh if the
circumstances weren't so desperate. I just hope that they
both understood I had no interest in blame or letting out
my emotions on anyone, but only in trying to figure out the
best way forward. No part of me wanted to be screaming,
'Well, this is an absolute bloody outrage and what are you
going to do about it?' at anyone. I wanted to be able to help.

I replied:

Well done. And just so you know, the Sun newspaper
has the details of you being in hospital. And it's lovely
because you're getting hundreds of messages of
support for you, which I want you to know about – from
everywhere! I'm desperate to speak to a doctor or
anyone. Please keep prompting them to call.

He sent a picture of him in a mask giving a thumbs-up with
an anaesthetist.

I'm absolutely desperate for this induced coma to
happen, if it's possible and they can get ventilators. If
you can speak to them, please ram it home, I cannot
take it any more, the constant feeling of drowning. The

lovely anaesthetist says it is very safe. But they want
to wait.

I bombarded him with questions, thrilled he was replying
to messages:

Why are they telling you they don't want to put you in
the coma? I know it's torture, but they are telling ME it's
better if you can keep conscious for as long as possible
because the ventilators can be so traumatic if they are
forcing your lungs open and closed while unconscious.

And I will never forget his reply:

It's Hobson's Fucking Choice. More damage while
unconscious or this slow drowning, like I am suffocating.
I love you so much, I know you are trying to save me,
but I just can't breathe – it's mental torture. I need a
break. I want to be put unconscious.

I couldn't let him know that I felt as if a cold pebble had
just dropped into the pit of my stomach; I had to make use
of every moment. I hit him with a paragraph of questions
about hydroxychloroquine and steroid treatments. My late-
night research online had been intense. I then listed names
and messages from everyone who had been in touch with
me, from my workmates to his former colleagues Peter
Mandelson and Tony Blair, each of them sending love, telling him he was a fighter and so on.

> That's so lovely give them my love too. Let's see what
> the night brings. Lovely to get these messages from
> people. Kiss Yems. Trying to get some sleep now.

'Yems' was another family word coined by Billy, who couldn't say 'them' for a long time and said 'yem' instead, so 'Yems' was Derek's nickname for the kids.

I texted back:

> I love you very very much. Keep going I am on it.

A friend of Derek's, Ben Wegg-Prosser, had seen he was sick in the papers and texted him immediately. Derek texted back (the only person he had managed to respond to directly apart from me) saying thank you and could he look after me. Ben texted me, wondering if he could help.

Ben is one of Derek's oldest friends and I had met him many times but in fifteen years I'm not sure we had ever spoken directly without Derek being there – we'd certainly never shared anything personal, just exchanged general niceties. He had never struck me as emotional. Sensitive and caring, yes, but definitely not someone who expressed it with flailing and wailing. Maybe this was just what I needed. By now I was being deluged with calls, from close friends and family, by friends of Derek and from other wonderful people. It was so touching and helped me feel less alone, but I was focused on saving Derek and conscious of keeping the line free, plus I wanted to keep Derek's mum and dad in the loop on everything, so I didn't have a second to respond to anyone.

Also, although I didn't realize it, I was also getting sick with Covid and was totally exhausted. I knew I needed support and there was something about Ben's direct, practical text that made me call straight back.

'Right, Ben,' I said, dispensing with any small-talk. 'He's in a bad way, struggling for breath. It's almost impossible to get through to the hospital and I can't visit either. I need to speak to someone senior, see if he can and should be put on a ventilator and what else can be done. Please help me to cut through.'

'Right. On it,' he said.

It was music to my ears. I immediately sent Derek another text:

> OK, we've got our own Derek COBRA going on now,
> like the one the government has for Covid!

I hoped he'd love the idea that a team was coming together, be reassured I wasn't battling alone:

> We're making calls behind the scenes, not in a pulling
> strings kind of a way because that isn't how it works,
> just trying to make sense of things. If you can get a
> message to someone please say we are trying to speak
> to the consultant in charge of your care. Please tell him
> it's just for five minutes. I'm obviously trying my end
> but if they come to you ask.

The reply arrived:

> No one's come to me in three hours.

I responded:

> God, you have no idea how good it is to get that text
> even though it's a horrible one. I can now actually get
> some sleep. It's 1 a.m. Darcey is cleaning the family
> room in a demented way – actually causing more chaos
> than good. But it's obviously okay.

I thought it might help to hear a bit of normal domestic stuff from home. Then I added:

> Don't worry, she's made everybody promise not to
> touch the pictures on the fridge!

Derek always insisted we never remove any of the children's paintings, done when they were much younger and brought home with pride from nursery. They often drove me mad, the paper peeling away from the fridge, being brushed askew as I hurried past them. Magnets could barely cope with the volume of brightly coloured but indistinguishable squiggles and swirls, and I had often expressed a longing to tidy things up a bit. But Derek loved them: they represented family to him. Only we remembered the meanings of those pictures, which had been there since the day they came home, and to move them would be to hurry past a bit of their childhood. So they had stayed, curling softly away from the cool white of the fridge-freezer, like posters for Derek's love for his family.

But instead of the warm response I was hoping for, a sign he had taken some comfort from my text, his return hit a much more desperate note:

> Babushka [one of his silly names for me] I don't think you realize how bad it is. It's utterly, utterly grim. I have to take it literally one second at a time. I'm still locked into the mask non-stop apart from about ten seconds every two hours to sip water. It is unimaginable. I literally feel like I'm drowning and I think every breath is my last. Please tell them both I love them. The doctor says there's no chance of me dying. I just have to keep going.

It was heartbreaking to read, but those words *no chance of me dying* shone out like a beacon. Were they true? Was there real hope?

I immediately fired off a string of messages back, sympathizing with his torture, encouraging him to keep going, telling him that I believed in him and that everyone was fighting for him. I stared at the screen, gazing at the trail of blue bubbles from me, hoping to see a white one from him ping back. But there was nothing. No news, no response. Nothing.

The nothingness broke with a phone call from Dr M in the very early hours. And it was obvious from his seriousness that it wasn't the news I had been hoping for. 'I thought we were going to lose him this evening,' he said. 'Because we just couldn't get his blood-oxygen levels up, however much we forced into the breathing apparatus. We were on near 100 per cent oxygen going into the mask and levels are still dropping in his bloodstream. Also I am very concerned about his kidneys. They are clearly under duress and failing. We want to get him on dialysis so we're also locating a machine for that. I'm worried about his liver and heart too. But for now our greatest priority is his lungs: we have to get more oxygen in. I think we have stabilized him a bit now but we need to see how the next few hours go.'

I felt sick, barely able to take in the detail, just hearing that he was slipping away, slipping away.

I had absolute confidence in Dr M's ability, but once again was struck by the awful sense of foreboding that if someone as qualified as he was, an expert in his field, was telling me that things were this bad, there was no escaping it, no explaining it away. Each time I had tried to call the hospital I prayed I wouldn't have to speak to someone who didn't sound sure, who didn't know what they were doing, who seemed inexperienced, but a tiny part of me would have found comfort in that. I could tell myself, 'Maybe they were too inexperienced to know. Maybe they weren't familiar with Derek's case.' I could keep wondering if someone more experienced would think of something to help. But with Dr M I was at the end of the line: with him, there was no 'Can I speak to your manager?' If he couldn't offer hope, maybe there wasn't anything else that could be done. I couldn't accept that. I couldn't give up.

I think I drifted off, then came to on the phone and realized he was still talking, phrases like 'Wait and see' and 'We doctors are learning more about Covid all the time' and 'In the next few hours we'll know more.'

Cutting across his attempts to be comforting I asked flatly, 'What happens if you can't get his oxygen levels up?'

'Well, we're moving towards putting him into the induced coma, which will give his lungs a rest and we can, put bluntly, force more oxygen in.'

'And what happens if that doesn't work? I mean, what's the plan next?'

He paused.

'There must be something,' I said. 'What about the hydroxychloroquine? I've been reading that it can be given with the antibiotic azithromyacin, and my friend Carla says they have been getting favourable results in LA. And steroids?' I was getting into my stride now. 'Certain steroids like dexamethadine?"

'Dexamethasone,' he corrected gently.

'Yes, that's the one, dexamethasone! I hear it can reduce the inflammation Covid causes and control the body's immune response, which I think some doctors are now realizing can cause as much damage as the virus itself. And what about antivirals? My friend who has had Covid and is now better says he took them and it made a world of difference and he says he can get me some … Would that help?'

I must have sounded a bit crazy, scraps of information from Google, from news reports, from mates of mates. He could have said, 'Leave it to the experts, love.' But he didn't. He continued.

'Listen, Kate, these treatments can only be used in the NHS as part of formal trials, and not all hospitals are doing trials. We haven't even been legalled to start them yet. The only one we are doing is the hydroxychloroquine."

'Well, put him on that,' I begged. 'I've already talked to him and he's up for trying anything that helps. He's just desperate to feel something's being done to ease his torture – he even wants to go into the coma, just for relief.'

He responded wearily. 'I know, I know. I've talked to him – he's begging for it. And as for the experimental treat-ments, within the NHS these can only be given as part of recognized trials. I know you and he want to be part of those so have put him forward. But I'm afraid I have more bad news. The selection for trial is randomized. We doctors do not get to choose. It's a computer that decides who gets the real medicine and who goes into a second control group and gets a placebo medicine. And I am afraid Derek has come out in the control, which means even if we get the go-ahead to start the trials he won't get any real medicine.'

'*What?*' I almost screamed, feeling waves of panic rising. 'But that's almost immoral. You've said yourself this is like fighting a war – you don't give someone in a trench a fake painkiller for a battle wound just to find out what painkillers work best in the future. This is a crisis. Please, for the love of God, give him what he needs!'

'Kate, it's not as simple as that. We have no idea if these drugs work – or, worse, if they might actually cause more harm than good. Other countries may do it but there is a reason why the NHS has rules about who gets what and when.'

He was right, of course, and deep down I knew it. Much later, I would find out that, tragically for Derek, some of the things I was suggesting would have helped, reducing the damage Covid inflicted. But back in March, when no one really knew what the virus was or what it truly did to the body, the medics were forced to treat the symptoms as best they could with knowledge from other diseases. It would have been a game of Russian roulette to chuck everything at Derek's already failing body, a game that might just as easily have killed him as saved him.

'There must be something, though, Doctor,' I pleaded. 'We can't just let him die.'

'There is one process but it's brutal. It might keep him alive, but it carries with it huge risks, and it's certainly not a cure.'

'What is it?' I asked, reaching for a pen and paper.

'ECMO – extracorporeal membrane oxygenation. Put simply, it bypasses the lungs. We would literally pump Derek's blood out of one leg, fill it with oxygen and pump it back in the other. He would have to be in an induced coma for that. We don't do it at this hospital and there are strict criteria about who gets it. He may not qualify. But I can look into it if you want and start to do the paperwork.'

I could hear the exhaustion in his voice – the long shifts, the weariness of having constantly to deliver bad news, the endless fight he feared he was losing. 'I should let you go, Doctor. You need to get some sleep.'

'I'll call you as soon as I know more. You should get some sleep too, Kate.'

But there was no way I could sleep. Adrenalin was coursing through my veins. The first flickers of dawn were creeping through the window. All I could think was that I had to be ready, at all times, for the paperwork, for giving authorization, for reading up on anything that might help. Thankfully the children were sound asleep. I crept around the house, unable to keep still.

Got to save Derek. Got to save Derek. Got to save Derek went through my mind over and over again.

And something else. Something dark, ugly. Something almost primeval, like a monster from the deep surging up, roaring. I had been crushing it down since the day Derek had first got sick. This time it was not going to be squashed. I couldn't hold it in any longer. I grabbed a cushion and buried my face in it to muffle the howl of *It's not fair!* Why did *he* have to get sick? Why did he have to get *so* sick when others had recovered? Why did it have to be someone who just wanted to be with his family? Why should he be stripped of everything, robbed of seeing his kids grow? Why did he have to be the one to miss out on the trials, to miss out on drugs that might have helped?

The ball in my stomach was like a hot fist of fury now.

What about me? Why should I be left here on my own? We were so happy! Why? Why? Why him? Why *him*?

Then … Why didn't I see it coming? Was it my fault? Did I miss something? God, if it's my fault, why not punish me? Why punish *him*?

I was almost in a daze now and, without realizing, found myself at the top of the house, a tiny room in the attic, no more than a cupboard, really. An awkward space that was too small to be turned into anything useful, like a bedroom, but Derek called it his Thinking Room. He used to go there to ponder something tricky he was puzzling out for work, to meditate or just take time out when life got on top of him. Having studied psychology later in life, he took his mental health seriously and enjoyed having this tiny space in the house to go and just be.

In our time together, Derek had taught me a huge amount about what our minds can do for our bodies, and how powerful our thoughts and positivity can be for us. He had come out of the darkest time of his life, a full emotional breakdown after years of depression and leaving a career in politics, to retrain as a psychotherapist. He had changed lives with his practice, and had certainly changed mine, not just as a partner but as someone whose outlook had taught me so much about getting through difficult times. As I sat up there in his space, I tried to focus on positivity, to think about how strong Derek was and how much he had already survived. I tried to think about how many of us there were on his side, the top-class doctors looking after him, and how lucky we were to have them.

As I looked around the room I suddenly saw how he had made it his own in his very Derek way. It was scattered with incense burners and room sprays with labels saying 'Pure Love' and 'Chakra Cleansing'. He had a bowl of sand he had taken from a beach in Cornwall that we both loved. I had seen him running his hands through it while he sat there. I ran mine through it too. It was calming, like fiddling with worry beads. Straight in front of me was a large brightly coloured wall-hanging of the young Buddha, meditating, and little statues of him too. He had a statue of Jesus, a crucifix, and a collection of Hindu and Islamic pictures as well. All crammed into this tiny space. Typical Derek, I thought. Why bank on just one God when you can keep all bases covered? That made me laugh, which relaxed me and made me feel closer to him too.

Then I saw a photo of Derek and me on one of our first holidays together at Lake Como in Italy. He was standing knee deep in water, all beaming smiles with his big white belly and baggy shorts soaking wet. I was much lower in the water, at his elbow level, partly because I was a full foot shorter than him, even standing up straight, and also because I was clearly trying to hide my big white belly below the water line. I laughed at how ridiculous a pair we looked, and how incongruous that daft holiday snap was, stuck in the middle of Derek's man-cave of spirituality and contemplation. It was just so, well, normal.

Another thought stopped me in my tracks. Normal. How many other people were doing just what I was doing right now, gazing into the eyes of a loved one, separated from them by this ghastly virus? How many others were praying they would come through? Worse still, how many more had had their beloved ripped from them?

I shouldn't be asking, Why Derek? After all, these other people, thousands and thousands of them, all had their version of Kate, who loved them, Darcey and Billy, mums, dads, brothers, sisters, lives they wanted to live.

I should be asking, Why not Derek? He was no different from anyone else. Just because he was special to me, there were thousands of others special to their loved ones. Love didn't make anyone safe from Covid. And, after all, he was still alive. He still had a chance.

I started to feel waves of gratitude for the doctors and nurses who were caring for him, for the system in which he could be cared for. I was grateful a hospital was close enough when we needed it, for the friends and family around us, for the hope he could still make it through.

'Thank you, thank you, thank you,' I was muttering under my breath, almost like a mantra. I was calmer now, the anger gone. I went downstairs, made a cup of my favourite strong builders' tea and curled up on the sofa, grateful too that my beautiful children were safe and still asleep. I tried to drift into an exhausted sleep myself.

I must have dozed off because I was still there at six in the morning when the call came.

'Hi, I'm with Derek now on speakerphone,' said a doctor whose voice I didn't recognize, on call before Dr M arrived. 'We're going to put him into an induced coma shortly so now is your chance to speak to him.'

'What, *now*?' I asked, sitting up and kicking the rug off my lap. My heart was racing anew.

'Yes.'

'OK.'

The next voice I heard was Derek's.

'I love you,' he said. 'You saved my life. And I don't just mean now because I'm going into the coma to help me. I mean, everything, with the children, the family, our wonderful life. You saved me.'

'I love you too,' I said, calling the kids' names to wake them up so they could speak to him too. 'It's just for a few days, to give you a rest, but keep fighting, keep going. We all believe in you and are taking care of you.' I was breathless now and the words were tumbling over themselves as I scrambled up the stairs to give the kids the phone.

'Wait, wait!' I almost screamed. 'Here's Darcey and Billy to say I love you.'

'Stop, Kate,' said the stranger's voice. 'He's gone under. He can't hear you. We'll call you later when he's settled, but we have to go now.'

The line went dead.

I slumped down on the stairs, glad the children hadn't woken up.

The nothingness and silence of the phone, still glued to my ear, was deafening.

I was alone, achingly alone. Would I ever hear his voice again? Then another voice I like to think of as Derek's came into my head: Right, Garraway, this is not the time to sit around. Crack on.

I looked at his picture on the wall and said out loud, 'I am here, Derek. We are going to get through this. You are alive, and while there is life, there is hope.'

Right, I thought, standing up and almost literally shaking myself down. What next?

Chapter 3

Joy

The morning I first heard the name Derek Draper was so spectacular that even a romance novelist might have thought it a bit much for the day I found out about the love of my life.

It was 2004, back in the days when I was working on *GMTV*. One summer morning the then political editor Gloria de Piero and I were heading down the stairs from the newsroom to the studio in ITV's former building on the South Bank in London. We used to call that old building Telly Towers as it was a twenty-four-storey skyscraper, and *GMTV* occupied three floors. The staircase was on the outside of the building and had floor-to-ceiling windows facing east overlooking the river Thames, St Paul's Cathedral and beyond. It was perfectly placed for seeing the sun rise over the landmarks of London. It always felt like a lucky morning if your trip from the newsroom to the studio was timed just perfectly to catch the magic light, and that morning was one of them: dawn was breathtaking, beams of light projected across the clouds, a golden glow making the river sparkle and the glass of London's skyscrapers flash. It reminded me of old religious paintings, as if it were my very own Botticelli, and I almost expected to see cherubs and angels floating on the pink and yellow clouds ahead.

Gloria and I were chatting away when she suddenly stopped dead and grabbed my arm so abruptly I almost fell over. Then, eyes wide, she said in her thick Bradford accent, 'Oh my God! I'm having an epiphany! You and Derek Draper! You'd be perfect together!'

'Who is Derek Draper?' I asked.

'Don't you worry about that,' she told me, as she started walking again. 'You're going to love him. He's so much fun. I'll sort everything out.'

I was single at the time so was used to friends' well-meaning attempts to set me up on 'dream dates'. They were always good fun but so far hadn't led to any happily-ever-after. So I only half listened that morning as she regaled me with tales of 'brilliant Derek' all the way down the stairs and as we were being 'beautified' in Makeup. All her stories seemed to involve him wildly partying, buying whole groups of people champagne in the Groucho Club. The Groucho is a legendary club in London famous for attracting acting and media types. At that point I'd heard of it but never been to it. Back when Derek and Gloria would go to it, it was most famous for being the epicentre of 'Cool Britannia', the sort of place you would find famous actors chatting with supermodels. Other stories seemed to focus on Derek getting into various mild scrapes and blagging his way out of them, chatting up girls 'way out of his league' but always winning them over so that they fell totally in love with him.

It was definitely not the sort of thing that impressed me. I had been hurt many times in relationships and would have been much more impressed with tributes of loyalty and kindness. He did not sound like my type at all.

'He sounds like a bit of an idiot, Gloria,' I ventured, not wanting to crush her enthusiasm.

But she beamed back, undaunted. 'Oh, he is! He's a total idiot. But also a genius. He's got a heart of gold and is completely adorable.'

There was clearly no stopping her, and we were getting closer to going on air for *GMTV*. I wanted to get back to rereading my notes and the briefs on the guests we had coming on the show, so I simply gave her a limp 'Great!' and thought little more about it.

Unbeknown to me, Gloria was now on a mission to get us together.

I don't know what made her quite so sure that this masterplan would work out, because on the face of it Derek and I are very different. He is six foot two and almost professionally northern, so proud is he of his Chorley roots. I am five foot two, from the home counties, and have no view on the Wars of the Roses. If you're from Yorkshire or Lancashire you'll already know what I mean by this. It seems that every time people from the two counties get together, especially when alcohol is involved, the Wars of the Roses crops up. Anyone from anywhere else looks on mystified.

Although very interested in politics and how it impacts on all of us, I have never been party political and certainly never been a member of any political party. From the age of nine or ten Derek had been reading party manifestos and was determined to revolutionize the Labour Party, which led him to be part of the movement to bring in New Labour. Back then he even had a picture of Roy Hattersley, now Baron Hattersley of Sparkbrook, one of his modernizing heroes, on his bedroom wall, while other people his age had Kylie Minogue or Kate Moss. I would tease him about this mercilessly, saying what a political nerd he was. He would always respond, 'You should be grateful, darling. Those were my formative sexual years when my hormones were raging and I woke up to Roy's face! However ropey you look in the morning you're always going to be gorgeous compared to him!'

Despite our constant teasing and banter, I have always been proud of Derek's desire to stand up and be counted politically. His spirit and drive to change the world for the better ran through him to the core. I was so glad that his colleagues from that time treasured it too. Some of the most touching messages I have been getting since he has been sick are from people he knew in those intensely political days, saying how much he had achieved for others. And they were coming from all sides of the political fence, from people who didn't necessarily agree with his views but appreciated that he was working for something he believed in, just as they did.

Derek has always been larger than life, loud and rumbustious, working hard and playing hard, all of which made him great fun to be around. Not that he didn't rub some people up the wrong way – in his political life he definitely understood that you can't make an omelette without breaking eggs. While I am the sort of person who walks into a lamp-post and apologizes to it, his political mates always said he would relish his verbal dust-ups with the opposition, the press and even his colleagues.

But there was another side to him that his close friends, like Gloria, knew was as strong as his fighting spirit. They had been good friends since she was a teenager, and she too had been a part of that world, as a member of the new Labour Party when she was a student. Because Derek was older and more experienced than her, she had always looked up to him politically. So Gloria knew about his fierce loyalty to the people he cared about, his generous spirit and, despite his outgoing partying ways, she had sensed he was a family man at his core.

She also knew he had been through a hugely difficult time in his life, having endured a breakdown and a period of depression, which had led him to turn away from London and his career in politics and head to Berkeley, California, to study psychology. Now, after four years, he was back with his master's degree, ready to set up his own psychotherapy practice. Gloria and he had recently met for lunch to catch up and he was buzzing about his plans.

Maybe that was what had lodged Derek in her memory bank so that she was ready to spring her 'epiphany' on me that *GMTV* sunny dawn. And I'm glad she took that shot with her Cupid's arrow. From time to time in the intervening seventeen years up to last spring she would send me a little text saying, 'Did I do OK, Kate? Did I do the right thing?' And I can say with an open heart that she absolutely did.

After that first mention of Derek, Gloria and I didn't speak about him again so meeting him was the furthest thing from my mind when, a month or so later, Gloria arranged a drinks party at Claridge's for a few of her friends, including a gaggle of our colleagues from *GMTV*. She invited Derek and me too. She told Derek it was a set-up but somehow he'd got the wrong end of the stick about who he was being set up with. He thought it was the stunning Andrea Maclean, best known now for her years on ITV's daytime show *Loose Women* but who was then *GMTV*'s weather presenter. He had googled her, seen how gorgeous she was, and was very excited about meeting her. Gloria didn't tell me Derek was going to be there and certainly not that *this* was a kind of blind date for us. Given that he thought he was meeting someone else entirely, and I had no idea who he was, when we did meet that Friday night, neither of us realized that we were already *on* our blind date when we started chatting.

It was a daft state of affairs, but also kind of brilliant. As far as I was concerned, I was chatting away to a lovely guy without the pressure of thinking I had been set up with him, and I suspect it made him more relaxed too, not realizing I was the one he was supposed to impress. I liked him immediately, and found him interesting as well as funny.

I remember thinking he had quite sad eyes, and it turned out I wasn't far from the truth. It had been the darkest of times that had led him to California. Now he would argue that that had helped him to grow in a way that made him more openly sensitive. He had been through a lot, and was just coming out on the other side. But, of course, I didn't know that because I was still waiting for my set-up to arrive, as was he.

After a while, Gloria came up and whispered in his ear, 'How's it all going?'

'Great. I really like *her* actually, so where is Andrea?'

'No, you idiot!' She slapped his arm. 'It's her – Kate – I'm setting you up with!'

I don't know what he said to her next, but within a little while the drinks were starting to peter out and Derek was talking about going to Mirabelle, Marco Pierre White's restaurant round the corner on Curzon Street. It had been a favourite of his gang back in the old days. Derek ostentatiously announced he could get us all in there without a booking as they KNEW him. Much later he confided he was trying to impress me, giving me a flash of the 'old Derek', but inside was panicking that he wouldn't be able to get us in. After all, it had been years since he had been there. Here was a first taste of the Derek bravado and the worried little boy inside who, over the next few years, I was going to come to know so well.

He needn't have bothered anyway. He didn't know it then but those flourishes always go right over my head. I wasn't impressed by fancy restaurants or that kind of pulling strings but I was pleased when he secured us a table as I didn't want the evening to come to an end. We were a smaller group by now, but full of laughter and giggles. Derek was holding court, entertaining us all with anecdotes, and we chatted some more. One of my friends was going through a hard time. She had recently split up with a boyfriend whom she'd thought she was going to marry, and she was still very raw about it. She was trying to put on a brave face but every now and then, especially as the alcohol flowed, bits of her pain would leak out.

'Oh God, am I just unlovable? What is *wrong* with me?' she burst out at one point.

We all rushed to reassure her there was nothing wrong with her, that he was an idiot, she was totally lovable and we all adored her. I noticed that Derek didn't speak but was just watching her carefully. She rallied with our support and got back into the swing of things. Later she said, 'I don't understand why I can't get over this. I feel so guilty about being destroyed by this one man. I know I'm so lucky really. There are people in the world who are fighting cancer, whose kids have died, there are people getting gunned down in wars – they have real problems. I feel so bad that I can't get over this.'

Before any of us could pipe up with more reassurance, Derek spoke. 'Of course you feel worse about what's happening to you. Why would you be as affected by strangers being gunned down in wars? You don't know them. That's not going to touch you emotionally in the way this man did. Even kids dying of cancer, why would you care about that?

Unless it's your kid, you aren't going to feel the same hurt as you do about what's happening to *you*.'

No one knew what to say. Hearing Derek dismiss children dying of cancer in such a blunt way left us all a bit stunned. But my friend looked slightly relieved. 'Doesn't that make me a bad person, though? Worrying about the feelings I have inside my head when other people have real tangible problems?'

'I have no idea whether you're a bad person or not. I don't know you. But I know that experiencing emotions that mean something to you doesn't make you bad. It's what you're supposed to do. Listen, what's happening inside your head is every bit as real as what happens in the so-called real world. Your emotions, your hurt, and the pain it's bringing up – that's real. Feeling guilty about it won't help. Acknowledging it, working it out and trying to learn from it just might …'

It was classic Derek: blunt, slightly disconcerting, different, but clever and insightful. It turned out it was just what my friend needed. Months later she admitted that what he had said to her that night was a real turning point for her, and that getting over the split had started right there, at that dinner.

I was intrigued. And as the evening ended and I headed home, I was pleased when Gloria texted to say that Derek had asked for my number. I hoped he would call.

Later that weekend he left me a voicemail. He sounded like he was speaking in a wind tunnel. I later found out he was on the Isle of Wight ferry visiting a friend, but the voicemail was so bad I couldn't make out his phone number to call him back. Fortunately, he called again a few days later.

'Oh, you do answer your phone sometimes, then,' was his cheeky opening gambit.

I explained why I hadn't called back. He sighed and said that on the answerphone message he had asked to take me out for a drink, and he had hoped to do so today, but that now he wasn't sure if we should go. He explained that a girl he had been very close to, and had had a relationship with in America, was getting married today.

'I just think it would be too weird, too pointed, to go on a first date with another woman the same day. I like you, Kate, and I don't want to have confused feelings when we're out together.'

O-*K*, I thought. Bit odd. After all, I hadn't agreed to go out with him and he could have chosen not to mention it, just arranged another time. Was he still hung up on this woman? Was I getting myself into a whole lot of trouble? But I was intrigued by his honesty. It was refreshing.

'So,' he continued, before I could respond, 'instead of seeing you, I've now arranged to help out at my church's amateur watercolour painting exhibition. You know, serving the cheese and wine, that sort of thing.'

A pause, while I wondered when the punchline was coming.

'But you can come along and help out with me if you want.'

There was no punchline. It was certainly the most random invitation I'd had in a while. Was it some sort of a test? It just seemed so preposterous! What had happened to Mirabelle, Claridge's, or perhaps a nice restaurant in a cosy corner of London? Derek's invitation seemed almost intentionally unglamorous. It was a world away from the stories of him whisking girls away to Paris and Italy that Gloria had told me. But something in me knew it would be a good idea so I said yes.

I showed up at the church, St Mary's in Primrose Hill, having struggled to find the right outfit for this weird date. Casual, practical, but with a hint of sexy? Who knew? There was still a part of me that thought it would *all* be a wind-up. That he would be standing outside the church with a bunch of flowers, about to whisk me off for a night out in the West End. But no, there he was behind a trestle table inside, in a salmon pink jumper, busy passing round the cheese and wine as people admired the local water-colour exhibition.

This was only the second time we had met, so I had no idea if there was something ironic or insincere about him wanting to help at his church. But now I know he *is* religious. When he had had his breakdown a year or so before, he had turned to Buddhism, Zen and all sorts of other faiths, but one of the books he had come across had had a quote from the Dalai Lama saying he had no respect for Westerners who turn to the religions of the East without first exploring and respecting the religion of their own country, born of their own cultural heritage. Derek was still working in Westminster at the time and one lunchtime walked into St Stephen's Chapel, within the Palace of Westminster, sat down amid its peace, and thought, *Yes* ...

Over time he had come to believe that learning about a variety of faiths is not about picking out the bits you like and ignoring the rest. But that if you study them even a little, you start to see how interconnected they all are. So, you should respect your cultural heritage and what its own religion offers before reaching to the East for mystical answers.

So there we were, in St Mary's Church, Primrose Hill, without a trace of irony. And do you know what? I loved it.

As we walked through the church a sign declared, 'By your deeds shall ye be judged.' We got married beneath it, and Derek continued to taunt me with that phrase at home for years to come.

'Aargh, I'm going to tidy up! I am!' I could be heard promising.

'*Weeeell*, by your deeds shall you be judged …' he would tease me.

Back then, I remember thinking that his jumper made him look like a little boy. It was the sort of thing I would put Billy in now and go, 'Ooh, this'll keep you nice and warm.' It most definitely wasn't the sort of thing I would have recommended a male friend wear for a first date. The fifteen-year-old me would have been appalled, but now I thought it was sweet and it made me think, Well, at least you're confident enough not to rely on your jumper to bring some personality to the evening. I, meanwhile, realized my 'hint of sexy' – very high heels – had not been a good call for a cobbled church floor, and was relieved to sit down for a minute away from the throng. I watched him smiling and chatting and thought, Well, he's either very confident or a serious oddball, as this is a very strange first date. I was right on both counts: he turned out to be a bit of each.

I was very, very late for our second date. I was working, and called him to say that I didn't know how long I would be, should we cancel? But he didn't want to. He said he'd cancel the restaurant and just cook at his place. I arrived there three hours after we were supposed to have met. Yes, *very* late. As he opened the door he said, 'OK, there is something you need to know about me – I'm all about expectations.'

'I did say I was running late!' I protested.

'But not by this much.'

Fair enough. For a moment I was worried I might have ruined things, that he would hold it against me. But instead of being sulky, he simply expressed his feelings and got on with the evening. At the time I had no idea what a big deal it was that he had attempted to cook for me – it's the only meal he has ever made, as he's definitely no cook. It wasn't the best meal I'd ever tasted, but was without doubt one of the most important evenings of my life. After we'd eaten we were listening to music when an Aerosmith song came on: *Don't want to close my eyes … I don't want to miss a thing.*

I was smiling at him goofing around when he grabbed my hand. 'Come on, let's dance.' He spun me around the living-room floor. He was staring at me hard in the eyes, singing along to the track as it continued. And he just didn't stop. I couldn't believe it. It was so, as my daughter would say, 'cringey'. I was squirming, making jokes, trying to look away. It was the most awkward thing. But he was undaunted and just kept singing straight into my eyes for the *whole song*!

'I could tell you had a real issue with intimacy,' he joked later. 'I thought, I'm just going to force her to connect with me, to break through it.'

And he was right to: from that night on, we were a couple. Everything seemed to accelerate, helped by a medical drama of my own. I had been getting backache, which was misdiagnosed as a strain. The pain got worse and I started to feel ill in a way I knew couldn't have been caused by muscle strain. One night Derek just snapped and said, 'Right, that's it. I'm taking you to A & E.' I was admitted immediately with a severe kidney infection, and ended up spending weeks in hospital. One of the scans showed I had a lump on my kidney, which they feared was cancerous. I needed surgery to have it removed so they could test to see if it was malignant. It was a frightening time.

Looking back, it helped us as a couple. If we had gone on simply dating, me arriving freshly fake-tanned, blow-dried and keen to impress, he might never have got to know the real me so quickly. But sitting there in a hospital gown, with unshaven legs and no makeup, ill and fearing for my life, I was stripped bare. That he still came to visit every day made me trust that he really cared. We started to share our deepest feelings and fears. Subjects like commitment, marriage and kids (things you're usually wary of bringing up on early dates) suddenly seemed comfortably on the table.

By the time I emerged from hospital, relieved that it hadn't been cancer, it was nearly Christmas, and things were very intense between us. Derek told me he knew he wanted to marry me, but privately was trying to work out if *he* was in the right place for it. He said he'd never planned on falling in love so soon after returning to the UK, that he'd thought he'd have a few years to set up his practice, to be in a financial place to settle down and raise a family. But he didn't want to lose me and feared that, because I was already thirty-seven, I wouldn't hang around. He also didn't want to waste my time. By now I had shared so much with him that he could see how important having a family was to me. He could hear my biological clock ticking even if I wasn't aware of it. So he decided to go for it.

He proposed in February 2005 in classic Derek fashion: romantic and ridiculous in equal measure. We had decided to go away together for the first time: a weekend break in Cairo, taking advantage of the out-of-season offers. Derek had arranged for us to have a couple's massage, and because the hotel was so empty, we ended up with a huge and luxurious spa room to ourselves. It smelt gorgeous – there were flowers everywhere and even the floor was sprinkled with rose petals. After our massage, we jumped into the huge stone jacuzzi in the corner of the room and sank into the bubbles. Bliss! Then Derek suddenly looked serious. 'What's wrong?' I asked. He lunged forward off the jacuzzi seat and on to one knee. He had miscalculated the depth at the centre, though, and was virtually submerged. He was spluttering and spitting out water, while his right arm flailed wildly behind him. It was a ridiculous sight and I burst into a fit of giggles.

'Quiet,' he choked. 'I'm trying to be romantic!' And I suddenly realized he was down on one knee for a reason, and his arm was flailing around because he was scrabbling to reach a ring box he'd hidden behind him.

'OK,' he said, as he gathered his breath. 'I'll cut my speech short. Will you marry me?'

'Yes!' I exclaimed. 'Now get up before you drown!'

We both burst into a fit of giggles, and then into tears at the emotion of it all.

He had been anxious that I wouldn't like the ring and was worried that he didn't have enough money to buy me something flash and expensive. So his best friend from way back, Henry Birch (who would be our best man), gave him some advice. Derek calls Henry his posh mate. Educated at Eton and the son of a diplomat, he and Derek had met in the Westminster House of Commons canteen (yes, they really do call it that!). At the time, Derek was working as a special adviser to Peter Mandelson and Henry was doing the same job for David Steel. Chalk and cheese on the outside, they hit it off straight away. Henry introduced Derek to a whole new way of life and pretty soon he was weekending in posh country houses and flying away for holidays at his new mates' summer homes in Tuscany. He loved it. Not least because he relished being the only working-class northern lad in this posh gang – he wore it as a badge of honour.

Derek would always say the upper class knows the best hacks for saving money and Henry's advice about our engagement ring was no exception. He told Derek to steer clear of big Bond Street jewellers because, he said, you end up paying extra for the famous name. Go to an auction house instead. You get much better quality jewellery for the money, especially if you avoid the bigger auctions at the weekend.

So on a wet Tuesday afternoon, Derek took himself off to try to snatch a bargain. He looked at all the rings in his price range and instantly fell in love with a diamond and platinum ring dating from 1932 – he was smitten by its unusual art-deco-style setting. He bid, won and was thrilled with the price, but afterwards started to worry about whether or not I would like it. After all, it was not a classic sparkler. Would I like the art-deco style? Some of his female friends pulled faces when he told them he had got it from an auction, because the jewellery would have been second hand. 'Yuk! I wouldn't want to wear a ring a stranger had worn. What if they'd died in it? Or the marriage had ended in divorce? It could be bad luck ...'

So he had the ring polished and purified in some kind of herbal salt-water mix to rid it of bad vibes. Derek needn't have worried. I *loved* it. It turned out we were both obsessed with art-deco design – one of the few things that *hadn't* come up in our hospital bedside chats! We have since filled our house with art-deco furniture and objects, bargains bought at auctions and second-hand sales.

I had been married before, so had already done the huge family white wedding, and would have been happy to go along with whatever Derek wanted: big, small, home, abroad, I didn't mind. But Derek was clear: 'We are having the whole shemozzle. Church, family, friends. My dream is the *Four Weddings and a Funeral* set-up – girls in big hats floating around on a sunny lawn.'

We began excitedly planning for a classic English wedding the following year, June 2006.

I think some of my friends were a little concerned. Derek was unlike anyone I had ever been out with before and we seemed so different. Unlike me, though, they hadn't seen all the sides of Derek that I had experienced through those intense months when I'd been sick.

My friend Piers Morgan, who was then editor of the *Daily Mirror*, took the mickey. He and Derek had crossed swords many a time when Derek worked in politics and Piers was a newspaper editor, but ultimately they got on really well. When Derek and I, newly engaged, arrived at an event together Piers took one look at me and said, 'Derek bloody Draper, are you kidding me? If I had known you had set the bar as low as *him* I would have had a crack myself!'

Derek wasn't insulted at all and we even quoted it on the menu cards at our wedding.

Some friends were worried that it all seemed so quick. They had been through the break-up of my first marriage with me and, even though the wounds were healed, they feared I was doing something rash. It seemed so out of character for me. I am always very cautious, agonizing over big decisions, analysing the pros and cons to distraction. Yet here I was, jumping into a lifetime commitment to this colourful character who, to them, seemed like a stranger.

I, too, had moments of doubt: not about Derek, but about

the dizzying nature of it all. From Gloria's dramatic first mention, to the bonkers first dates, to the intensity of fearing I had cancer … Was I caught up in a crazy fairytale, a romantic whirlwind?

Fate stepped in once again. In the summer of 2005 we found out I was expecting Darcey. We were both thrilled. 'Let's just get married now!' Derek exclaimed. 'I'll feel different if we wait till after the baby's born. I want the day to be about us.'

'But what about your dream of a big summer wedding?' I exclaimed.

'We'll just organize a big autumn one in six weeks instead – we can do it!'

And we did. We managed to find a hotel with an underground ballroom that had survived the Blitz so had retained its original art-deco features. And it was available! Perfect. Derek was keen for us to marry in the church he had been going to for so many years, the one where we'd had our first date. When we asked the vicar of St Mary's if he had any free Saturdays in the autumn, he said the only one he had was 10 September – the date we had met for the first time in Claridge's! That sealed it. It was meant to be!

It was a wonderful wedding – we were surrounded by family and friends. As a surprise, Derek got our friend Crispin, a songwriter who had been in a band called the Longpigs, to perform a special acoustic arrangement of 'our' Aerosmith song for when we were signing the register. We both laughed at how much I'd squirmed the first time Derek had sung it into my eyes. Then, as Crispin was singing, one by one, all our friends and family in the church began to sing along and by the end their arms were up in the air swaying as though at a rock concert. It was hilarious and wonderful all at the same time.

Gloria was beaming for the whole day. 'I did good, didn't I?' she said, as she squeezed my hand in a quiet moment. She truly did. When I gave my speech after the ceremony, I was keen to thank her for introducing us, as well as thanking absolutely everyone who had made our high-speed wedding possible. I wanted to thank all my friends and family for their fantastic support throughout my life, and to make sure to welcome my new family, the Drapers. I remembered everyone. Everyone apart from Derek, that is. As I sat down, he looked at me and said, straight-faced, 'You completely forgot to mention me.' Oh, no! The one I'd wanted to thank the most! So I stood straight back up and said to the gathered mass of smiling faces, 'And a huge thank-you to Derek. Who saved my life.'

'Aww,' said the room in unison, as half of us (including me) started crying.

Later, he would tease me: 'My God! Thank goodness I saved you. You were so far back on the shelf you were behind the dusty old out-of-date pickle jars!'

Cheek!

'Hey, I saved *you* right back. Do you think anyone else would take you on?' And we'd laugh.

But the truth is that he did save me in a way. Without a doubt, he changed the course of my life. We really worked to have the relationship that we did. Worked to form the marriage we wanted, the family we had both longed for, with conscious and loving decisions.

When Darcey and Billy arrived, Derek blossomed. He was born to be a father. He relished every moment and got stuck in right from the start, cutting their umbilical cords and being the epitome of a hands-on dad.

We were content just to be, to potter about our home, and would often lie in bed and think how lucky we were to have found each other. That sounds hideously smug – and don't get me wrong: things weren't perfect. We had as many rows as any other couple. My untidiness drove him crackers. And his constant need to tackle everything head on, battle things through, exasperated me.

'Arrgh!' I would scream. 'Can't you just let things go? Say the easy obvious thing for once? You know, make small-talk?'

He would always reply, 'I'm the grit in the oyster that makes our pearl, darling.'

And maybe he was right.

As the years went by we seemed to be a yin and yang that made our life together work. I could be strong when he needed me, and he would pick me up and be there when I needed him. We were different, yes, but maybe that kept our balance.

And now that he was absent, the balance was gone.

There was a strange sense of emptiness to that Sunday morning after I had said, 'I love you,' and he had slipped into a coma.

I looked around and felt numb. I picked up my phone

to text Derek, but there was no point. He wouldn't be able to read it. He had had the procedure he had been begging for, the one that all the doctors were saying he needed. As we understood it, this was his best chance. But still I was consumed by the feeling of absence. It wasn't just that Derek wasn't there, but the absence of him seemed huge, filling every corner of the house, every room I went into, every drawer I opened, every childhood painting that brushed against my arm as I made my way around the kitchen. From the little ornaments we had collected on our holidays to the art-deco furniture, they just flooded me with vivid memories of shared love, of how we had tried to build a home special to *us*. Suddenly they seemed almost ridiculous. The straw donkey from Spain only made sense if Derek was laughing about it, too. The second-hand furniture suddenly looked like a junk shop without Derek rubbing his hands along it.

This doesn't work without him! my mind screamed.

I tried to think of practical things to do, to focus on. But time seemed to be expanding and contracting in a way that made no sense. I didn't even know what hour of the day it was at any given moment, and I couldn't work out when meals or sleep or anything sensible was supposed to happen.

'It's just three or four days,' I told myself. 'It's just three or four days.' But I didn't know what three or four days meant any more, what it might even feel like to live through. So how could I console myself with that? There wasn't the space to think about my feelings, though: I had two children upstairs who needed me.

'They've put Dad into a deep sleep,' I explained to them. 'It's a good thing. It's to give his lungs a decent rest.'

I looked at their little faces. They were just fuzzy hair and warm pyjamas. They didn't get it at all.

'Right!' I said. 'Let's do something fun while we wait for Dad to get better. Who wants to go out on the trampoline?'

But before we even got out of the door the phone rang again.

Chapter 4

Life on Hold

———

Calls that come in with withheld numbers are always a bit disturbing, aren't they? Until that moment, the only people I knew who had ever called me from one were Ben Shephard and Jeremy Kyle. With them, I had made an arrangement that they would text me first to say they were about to call. Otherwise I would never bother answering as I would always assume that it was some strange person trying to sell me insurance, PPI or worse.

Now, though, withheld numbers held a new terror. These days, they were something else entirely: calls from the hospital. Someone phoning from a random ward to tell me big news. Possibly bad news.

So, when I saw a withheld number calling me, I answered it with a sense of dread. A voice said, 'Hi, I'm calling from the hospital. We've managed to find an opportunity. Derek has been accepted to a hospital where they conduct ECMO. It doesn't necessarily mean he'll get a place, but it does mean he'll be in the right vicinity if a place comes through.'

'How does that work?'

'Well, the ECMO team from the hospital are going to carry out the transfer, and they'll call you direct. We're hoping that this will happen at around seven p.m.'

'And how is he doing?' I asked.

'He's stable,' came the reply.

There was something very reassuring about hearing 'stable', especially after the shock of Dr M's phone call when he had said that Derek's oxygen levels were plummeting so dramatically. Yes, 'stable' sounded wonderful. But later, over the weeks and months, I learnt it often meant that the person I was speaking to was not authorized to give me any other information. Or that they were just keeping him alive, nothing else. Only later did I realize that the situation had been critical on occasions when I had been told he was stable.

This is a good thing. This is a good thing, I told myself. He's going to be near the treatment he needs, and I'll know by seven p.m.

I updated Derek's family, then went back to distracting the kids with some fun in the garden. I thought the hours until evening would seem endless but I didn't have to wait long before I heard from the team: it was less than an hour later that the doctor arranging the transfer called.

'I didn't expect to hear from you until much later,' I said.

'No, we're here earlier than planned,' he said. 'But I'm

afraid there's bad news. He is incredibly sick. He is not well enough to be transferred. He needs to be hooked up to the ECMO now.'

'Is that even possible?'

'Well, the only way we can do it is by taking him into surgery in this hospital, and we'll have to see if they have space in a theatre here. If so, we can attempt to do the procedure here. That could work, but I need to check.'

'OK.'

He called back later to say he had good news. They had space in a theatre.

'That's great,' I said.

'Yes, but in order to do it, I first need to run through the risks with you. The procedure isn't simple and, as I said, he is a very sick man. There is no guarantee that we will get him on to the ECMO machine, and there is no guarantee that he will survive the process or indeed the transfer to the other hospital. But we can't keep him here for long as the kit we have is temporary. He needs to be set up properly.'

'What are the risks?'

'Well, there's a risk of his heart stopping. There's a high risk of stroke. And as with any operation, there's a risk of something unexpected going wrong.'

'Will he feel any pain?'

'He won't know anything about it. But it won't be quick.'

'What choice do we have?' I asked. 'Is he going to die without this?'

'It's my honest medical opinion that, yes, he will die if we do not do this.'

'Well, it's not really a choice, is it?' I replied.

'OK. I'm going to do it now,' he said, gathering himself. 'It's going to take me a while. You'll obviously appreciate that everything is taking longer at the moment with all of the PPE we're wearing, which makes it even more challenging.

'But I will do it,' he continued. 'And I'll call you afterwards. It will be me who calls.'

I put my phone down, my mind swimming with thoughts of the task ahead. And this guy had sounded so young. I couldn't believe that this young, clearly tired man was having to make such huge decisions. It was one of many occasions on which I was stopped in my tracks by how extraordinary our nurses, doctors and hospital workers are.

He would have had layers of PPE on, and just moving around looked tough enough but to do such a challenging operation seemed almost impossible, trying to perform delicate procedures wearing thick gloves while visors and glasses steamed up. I had seen images on the news and online of how much the secured masks cut into the young, vulnerable faces as people tried to care for swathes of sick patients. I suspected that he had been at work since very early that morning, and, because so few people in the country were trained in these procedures, they must be stretched to the limit and beyond. I later found out that many were working thirty-six-hour shifts to get through the numbers of cases they were being presented with.

I looked at Billy, sitting cross-legged on the floor a few feet away, playing with his Lego. My God, I thought. That young doctor is somebody's son too. He was somebody's little boy once, and now he's being asked to save someone else's dad. He's not just doing this for Derek, he's doing it for everyone he can find hours in the day to treat. On top of that, he's operating on Covid-positive patients, potentially putting his own life at risk. And it's not just him. It's teams of people like him, up and down the country, in hospital after hospital, ward after ward. They're all doing this, people's sons and daughters, trying to save the lives of other people's mums and dads. Their bravery was overwhelming.

I knew that taking a Covid-positive patient into the operating theatre meant that the entire room would have to be deep-cleaned before and after the procedure. Would that hold up other operations? Was Derek's care putting other fathers, other sons at risk? Other mums? Other daughters?

I was a second or two from losing myself in a panic about the toll of looking after Derek, but I pulled myself back, reminding myself that I had to make Derek my only priority. I had to squish away the growing surge of guilt.

'Look, at last, this is a bit of luck,' I told myself. 'They've got to him, and they've got to him in time. He was very unlucky to get so sick. He was unlucky not to get on the trials. But this time, it's a stroke of luck. Please, please, let him get through this …'

The next few hours seemed like an endless wait. Eventually, the call came.

'He's through it.'

'Is he OK?'

'Well, his oxygen levels are really low. It was very, very tough getting him on to the ECMO because he's incredibly weak. The blood is now coming out of one leg, being infused with oxygen then pumped back into the other leg. His blood vessels will be under duress. There has been some bleeding while we tried to get him on to the machine, but we've got it pumping successfully now, and we've got him stable enough.'

I found out later from another healthcare worker that his heart had stopped during the procedure but they had managed to get it going again.

'Right, now we have to try and transfer him for more specialist care.'

The journey to the new hospital was about seven miles but the young doctor warned me that it could take them hours to get there, because once they were en route, they had to do everything with painstaking care.

I felt reassured that Derek was on his way, but as I hung up, I felt overwhelmed by his vulnerability. There he was, completely unconscious, at death's door, and with a group of total strangers. I imagined him in one of those hospital gowns that you're given when you're admitted, and it falling away in front of people he had never met, who didn't know who he really was, who could see only the sickness, not the man. Suddenly this most precious thing in my world was in the hands of this group of brilliant but totally unknown people.

The reversal in our roles seemed pitiful. Derek was a six-foot-two rock of a man, while I have always been a bit of a feeble shrimp. He was always the one who lifted things from the top shelf, carried the heavy shopping in from the supermarket, got the bulky bags from the conveyor belt at the airport. He made it all look effortless while I was flailing around in his wake. Now, he was lying there, the weak one, while I tried to gather my resources. The thought of his vulnerability weighed heavily on my heart, as did the knowledge that I was far from the only person in the country going through this that weekend.

Half of the country seemed to have no clue how bad things were getting in the hospitals, while the other half seemed to be either working on the sick, or worrying about them. Life on hold, in a horrifying limbo. Waiting for change, waiting for news, waiting for hope.

I could hear people outside, playing, enjoying the sunshine, as I sat there, phone in hand, wondering how to carry on. They have no idea, I thought. It's as if they're living in another world.

Push this out of your mind, I told myself. You have to snap out of it. And, with a gasp, I remembered I had to tell Derek's mother about the conversation I had just had. After all, I had just made an enormous life-or-death decision about her only son. How would I feel if another woman made a decision like that about Billy, or Darcey? How could I wait a moment longer before telling her? I called immediately and explained to her the decision I had made, and that he had come through the procedure. I was trying to tell as few people as possible, as each conversation like that took at least an hour, allowing for explanations, tears and fretful wondering about the future. It was emotionally exhausting, as well as being further time I wasn't spending with the children. Derek's parents took on the role of telling his sisters, leaving me to try to focus on an evening with the kids.

By the time midnight came around I couldn't bear the wait any longer. I decided to call the hospital he was travelling to: perhaps the staff there were in touch with the team who were in transit. It took me twenty-five minutes to get through, but I explained that my husband was being transferred to the ECMO unit, and was immediately put through to the ECMO nurse.

'I don't have his name anywhere or his records,' she said, as she riffled through forms and other documents. I could sense she was getting more and more harassed as I tried to explain the situation, my heart galloping as I imagined all the awful reasons they might have no record of him. Eventually we stopped talking at cross-purposes and she realized he had not yet been admitted.

'Aaaah! I didn't know his name! But I know a team is coming to us. We have everything ready, and they're nearly here.'

I just hoped that this was Derek and that he was still en route.

'Someone will call you,' she said. That promise again. The gratitude mixed with the trepidation again. The waiting again. It took everything I had not to let anxiety get the better of me at the thought of that journey, but I focused on the words 'nearly here' and tried to rest.

The call eventually came at two in the morning.

'Kate, it's me.' It was the young doctor.

'Is he still alive?' This was how I began all conversations. I felt if I knew he was still breathing, still with us, I could manage my emotions better to take in whatever other information was to come.

'Yes, he is. He is. It's taken a long time to get here as we were so worried about him. I wanted to get him in and get him established before I called you.'

'Thank you.'

'But, Kate, you have to know he's very, very sick. You need to know that he might not make it.'

'I know. I get that,' I said quickly. But the blood was roaring in my head at hearing those words out loud for the first time. If I was honest with myself I'd been fearing it since he'd got into the ambulance at home, but hearing someone put it to me so directly had an enormous impact. Until that point, I'd been able to tell myself my imagination was running away with me. But now it was a reality with which someone else was confronting me – the someone who was in charge of Derek's care.

'We have to get him on some medicine. We need to do scans of his whole body so that we can see what's going on in there. We need to see more clearly the state of his lungs, which they did not have the resources to do where he was. And we're going to scan him and X-ray him from top to bottom. Then, we'll have a much clearer idea of what we're up against.'

'Can you also see if you can get him on some trials?'

'I'll make sure everyone knows you want that.'

As soon as I put the phone down I tried to focus on the word 'medicine'. It had the hope of something that would help, a positive 'action' rather than a passive 'wait and see'.

He's in the right place, Kate. You've already worried about the possibility of him dying. It didn't help. Focus on what you can do. He still has a chance.

I crawled into bed next to the children and snuggled down but I didn't really sleep. I repeated the mantras to myself: *He's in the best place ... He's alive ... He's been lucky ... Now sleep and you can deal with the rest in the morning.*

The following morning, they were still running tests when I called. It wasn't until after ten that evening that another doctor called to update me. Finally, here was a dedicated person who would be looking after Derek. He was off the ward after a long shift, but ready to tell me what they had discovered.

'Is he alive?' Once again, I had to get that question off my chest first. The surge of fear and adrenalin was so all-consuming that I was unable to absorb anything any doctor was saying until that first question had been answered.

'Yes.'

'Right, let me get a pen and paper,' I said. And so began what became nearly a year's worth of notes, tracking Derek's journey day by day, test by test, call by call.

'He's incredibly ill. We need to keep him stable. The ECMO seems to be working so far. We have done a full range of scans. His lungs are solid with Covid infection. He is stiff with it. The membranes of his lungs are so infected that the lungs themselves literally cannot inflate and con-strict. They are just not able to function.'

That sounded bad enough, but the problems were far more widespread than just taking care of his lungs.

'His heart is a concern. The beat is irregular. We're treating him with medicines to stabilize that. His kidneys have failed, so he's on full dialysis. And his liver is failing. His brain seems clear from inflammation ...'

'What? Can Covid cause an infection in the brain?'

'We don't know. Nobody knows. Nobody knows what Covid can cause. But at this point it looks as if he doesn't have that.'

'What would it mean if he had inflammation in the brain?'

'He doesn't have it. And let's be glad of that. Let's just say you don't want inflammation in the brain.'

I could tell I was pushing him further than he wanted to go, asking for more than he wanted to tell me, but I couldn't stop myself. They were experts in hearts and lungs, in life and death. So while they were doing their job, using their mind-blowing skills to the best of their abilities, I was trying to use mine. In this case, I was trying to extract as much useful information as possible. It was clear the doctor was tired, that he must have had dozens of calls to make, and that he was trying to give me all of the facts. But it was also becoming clear that there was just so much they didn't know yet.

'But I thought you had medicines to help him now?'

'Kate. There is no cure for Covid. Derek's best chance now is incredible *care*. Think what his body is going through right now,' he said. 'Oxygen is being poured into him artificially through tubes in his legs by this machine. We have to give him anticoagulants because we need the blood to flow freely. It can't get stuck either in his body or in the machine. It's punishing to his vessels and these anticoagulants carry a risk because they can cause bleeding where we don't want it – like the brain. He has clots in his lungs. I'm assuming he didn't have clots in his lungs before.'

'No, we'd have known if he had. He had a scan quite recently.'

'Well, that's very interesting, as we're now sharing our findings with other hospitals and we are discovering that Covid can cause clotting. The worry about that is where else the clots are forming. He is incredibly sick. At the moment, I can't do anything other than just keep him alive.'

Alive. Just think about that word, I told myself.

'I know how hard this is. But we're facing a disease for which there is no cure, Kate, and which we're not medically prepared for. All I can do is use all of my skills and experience to keep him alive, and hope that the tide will turn. That is what we're doing for all our patients.'

'What about steroids? What about everything else?'

'You don't give steroids to someone with an immune system as compromised as Derek's. At the moment his immune system is doing all it can to fight off this infection. He is so fragile, Kate, so fragile. He's clinging to life by a thread. If we do *anything* to rock the boat ...'

I let out a gasp.

He must have realized he had gone as far as he could in making me grasp the reality of this precarious situation. His tone now changed. 'We just have to take it minute by minute, hour by hour.'

'But that's unbearable. What you're telling me is that at any minute he could die.'

'Yes. You need to understand that he might not make it. You need to know that he might die. You *have* to prepare yourself for that.'

I didn't start to cry. I don't know what noise I made. What can you say when someone tells you this? I knew that panicking would help no one. I knew that I didn't have anything even close to the expertise that this doctor did. In that moment, all I could think was that I might throw up. Right then, right there. That was all I felt capable of.

There must have been something in the sounds I was making that told him his message had been received.

'Look, I don't like having these conversations any more than you want to hear them, but I just think honesty is the best way to go. He's come this far. We've got him on the machine now. We've got him here.'

'We're going to get through today.'

'Let's go for that. I'll speak to you later once we've got more medicine into him.'

As the call ended I felt gripped as if by a vice. I couldn't breathe. I still felt unwell from Covid that I had contracted just after Derek. What if I got more sick? What would I do about the children? Once again, the thoughts were thundering past, faster than I could deal with any of them.

How could I prepare for this? To be told my husband was dead? They were telling me I had to get prepared but there is no preparation for the call that tells you that you have lost someone. This was the fate of so many Covid patients and the people who loved them. Little did I know then that, for many of us, the situation would be ongoing a year later. It seemed unimaginable to get through one minute. I went to the bathroom and threw up, thanking heaven that the children were asleep in bed.

They say that when you are at the point of death, such as falling from a great height, your life flashes in front of your eyes. Years ago, I interviewed a neurologist who explained to me that this phenomenon is your brain desperately searching its memory banks for an experience you have already had that might possibly prepare you for this moment. Your mind is scrambling to work out what is happening, what skills it has to cope and how it can find a solution while riffling through all the data it has accumulated from your life so far.

In that moment, on the cold of the bathroom floor, that was exactly how I felt. As if I were falling and falling, faster and deeper than I ever had. Then, suddenly, something deep inside me saw a fresh way to view the situation.

Kate, you can do this. You have something. You have the skills. It's what you do when you're on air and there's a breaking news story. You have to wipe your worries away and just focus on the most important task at hand, what you can control. This is the plan: compartmentalizing your head and working step by step. You need to focus on what Derek needs, not worry about what might happen that hasn't already happened. You need to take care of the kids and make them feel safe. That you *can* control, I told myself. You have spent years broadcasting live on TV, training yourself to force your brain to focus on one moment, the moment of live broadcast, and that moment only.

I remembered that those moments of intense broadcast felt almost like a physical exertion, a muscular effort to force the focus on to one single thing. And that was what I had to do now.

OK, what does Derek need? I asked myself. He has the best possible care now. You can do nothing to improve that. What *do* you need to do? You are ill, and you are in the house in sole charge of two children. They are going to wake up at some point. And they are going to need you to be getting well, not sicker. I went to bed, whispering to myself, *He's got the best care. I can do nothing but sleep and be strong. He's got the best care. I can do nothing but sleep and be strong.*

That was the first time I realized I had already learnt skills I could use to try to help move the situation along. And, boy, was I going to need them.

Since that day, I have learnt that the doctors who were with him said he was the sickest Covid patient they had ever seen who hadn't died. They have many ways of assessing how badly someone is infected by Covid. One is to measure an enzyme the liver produces to tackle infection. A healthy person would be 10 or under. If you've got a cold you might be about 50, and when you get to 200, it's starting to look bad; 150 is the sort of rate you would have with bacterial pneumonia and you need to get to hospital sharpish. When Derek came on to the ward his enzyme rate was 1627. They said it was off the scale compared to anything they had seen in anyone who had survived. In their minds this was some-one who was going to die. They feared he would, all of them.

So, when they were preparing me, that was what they thought was going to happen. In the past, I had tried to take comfort from the fact that doctors always prepare you for the worst. It's part of their training. No one wants to be the doctor standing with a grieving relative who is saying, 'You told me everything was going to be OK!' They always have to prepare you for the worst. That was how I had been trying to reassure myself as I heard them telling me to be prepared. Only later did I realize they thought he really *was* dying. That was what they were steeling me for.

The next few days were a blur of trying to speak to someone at the hospital and, in between, living minute by minute. When I rang and managed to get through, I would always ask, 'Is he still alive?'

'Yes,' a voice would say.

OK, we've made it through another few hours, I would think.

Alongside this there would always be a drama to report. His blood-sugar levels would plummet, then surge. His oxygen levels would drop and there would be fears that they were losing him, or about the damage that lack of oxygen to the brain might cause. Then they would manage to get the levels back up, I would feel some relief, and they would try to reassure me that the levels hadn't been low enough for long enough to do any damage. None of it was fully reassuring, though, because all the while I knew that at any minute they could lose the desperate fight.

I would try all sorts of different questions: I had details of blood pressure, heart rate, enzyme levels, how much food he was absorbing through the tubes they were using to feed him. I was asking them about weight loss and they would say he was stable, it was going down or he had gained a little. It was a constant measuring of something it was impossible to measure – his chance of living – but it was just my way of trying to manage through fact something I knew even the doctors couldn't tell me.

Once I asked, 'How long can he stay on ECMO for?'

I heard a sigh on the line. 'Well, we only have previous occasions where we have used ECMO for other illnesses. Usually within two or three weeks, if people are going to show signs of improvement, they have done.' I immediately did a calculation. And the person I was talking to clocked that. 'Listen, Kate, it's early days. It takes the body a while to settle.'

Eventually, it became two weeks, then three.

'Where are we now?' I asked.

'We're just going to carry on,' they said. 'We're just going to carry on.'

I pleaded with them. 'Don't ever switch it off, will you? You won't just stop?'

'We are *not* going to give up on him,' they told me.

Whenever I had got through to the first hospital Derek had been in, it had been mayhem – like there was a football match going on in the background. But this ward was eerily quiet when I called. Of course it was: it was full of patients who were unconscious. I had such a clear vision of all of those beds: row after row of patients fighting for their lives, silently, but alongside each other. A terrible, eerily soundless battle.

I was aware that the staff there were having to do for each of the patients in those beds what they were doing for Derek, and it was horrible, overwhelming to think of the scale of the fight.

As time went on, I became increasingly aware of what pressure this battle must have been putting on the rest of Derek's body. For example, by now he was fully Type 1 diabetic, meaning that Covid had an effect on his pancreas to the point where it was not producing insulin. They were therefore having to manage insulin in someone who was unconscious. I was constantly trying to think of new questions to elicit information. Anything I could grasp at to help me prepare, to help me get a handle on things.

'Let me ask you this. How many people with Covid have you had come off ECMO?' I tried at one point.

'We have thirty machines here. They are all in full work. And so far we have had three successfully come off it. They're not as sick as Derek, but let's all just pray that he'll be the fourth.'

I didn't dare ask how many hadn't made it. I just had to focus on Derek being the fourth.

But another part of me was determined to keep on asking, to know as much as possible, to keep up my mission to stay informed, to keep motivating everyone. Because if I didn't, who else would? I was only looking out for Derek, but the doctors had ward after ward of people they were trying to save.

We got through each day. Slowly, agonizingly slowly, Derek's time on ECMO continued. Everything felt so static, the whole world on hold. No schools, no shops, not even any traffic on the roads. A huge pause button had been pressed on everyday life, but while it felt as if the rest of the world was learning Mandarin and the art of baking sourdough, our family was on pause too. Waiting for news, waiting to know, waiting to exhale.

While we were waiting, Derek's body was fighting. But, as with all epic battles, it was causing enormous damage. The strange nature of Covid-19 is such that, as bad as the virus is, the massive immune response it provokes also leaves a huge mark. As the body tried to fight, the side-effects were mounting.

Each morning the key team at the hospital would have a conference call with other hospitals across Europe, Spain and Italy particularly, as they had been the first to be hit very badly. What they were starting to understand was the nature of these secondary problems, especially in Bergamo, Italy. So it was that a day or two later they called to say that they were now learning about patients there who had been in the same situation that Derek was now in, and the issues were the same: inflammation in the tissues throughout the body and blood clots. Covid was causing blood clots in the lungs, and in the brain too. And this in turn could cause strokes and bleeds on the brain.

After a few more days of keeping Derek alive on the ECMO machine, the team called to say that they were going to give him a CT scan to check for further impact from Covid on his body. An MRI scan, which would have given them better and more information, was out of the question for as long as he was physically attached to the ECMO, but they wanted to use the best they could as soon as possible.

More waiting. More endless, perfect sunshine. More standing on the pavement, clapping for the NHS. More trying to coax the children into believing that, yes, it was worth doing their home schooling, even if life as they knew it was falling apart around them. Then came another definitive call. One I shall remember for ever.

'We have looked at a CT scan of Derek's brain. We don't know what it is, but something on the scans suggests that he may have had either a bleed on the brain or ... there are multiple little dots that could be multiple little clots. And clots mean a stroke.'

My heart obviously fell through my boots. 'What does that mean?'

'Well, it means we're seeing the impact on Derek's body in his lungs. We're seeing severe impact in his kidneys, his heart, how blood is moving around the body. And we may now see an impact on his brain. We don't know whether it is or isn't. In a normal situation we would take him immediately for an MRI scan and that would give us clarity on what's going on in his brain. But if we did that we'd have to take him off ECMO. And if we take him off ECMO he will die. So we just have to keep going. People can recover from clots. People can recover from bleeds. But if he comes off ECMO, he dies.'

Where there is life, there is hope.

This sentence flashed across my mind as I clung to the

possibility that Derek could survive those clots if only he could stay alive. It was a sentence that sustained me over the weeks and months that followed.

Where there is life, there is hope.

'You have to keep him on the ECMO,' I said.

'Yes, we do,' came the reply.

Once again, I was ending a phone call feeling as if I was hanging on a precipice, not knowing if Derek was going to live or die, helpless to save him. This was not a place I could survive in alone. Thank God help was all around me: I just had to learn how to find it, and to reach out and grab it.

Chapter 5

Hope

When the pandemic first made its way into our lives, each of us had a different way of talking about the invader.

'This is madness! They can't *make* us stay in our homes – it'll never come to that!'

'They're just scaring us. It can't be real …'

'It's like a Hollywood movie – the beginning of a Will Smith blockbuster when no one *in* the movie knows what's coming, but the audience does. We just need Will to save the day!'

My friend Lorraine Kelly, the ITV presenter, said she felt as if she was in a science-fiction movie, as if aliens had taken over the world.

None of us could find *quite* the right description from their own life to sum up the sense of unreality and fear we felt. Time and again we turned to the language of film, the world of fantasies seeming to give us the language that the real world couldn't.

In the first few weeks of the pandemic and lockdown the movie *Contagion* shot to the top of Warner Bros' download charts, second only to the Harry Potter franchise: people were looking for clues – wanting to find something in the movies that would help them prepare for what was happening. Or was it the sense that real life and the news seemed so unreal that fantasy and reality were blurring into one?

By April, I had my own movie running through my head. The only thing to which my feelings seemed to relate was *Alice in Wonderland*: a girl falls down a rabbit hole into a strange world. But my version wasn't the Walt Disney animation I'd watched as a kid, its bright colours and comical characters taking the edge off the terror. Instead at night I'd fall asleep and dream. I'd find myself in a horror-movie version of the *Alice* story in which I was falling, falling, falling and never hitting the bottom. The space was dark, but with just enough light for me to see twisted roots, like vines, around me. I reached to grab them and slow myself, arms flailing. But the roots were slippery ... like snakes, my pet fear. And suddenly the snakes were hissing at me so I was too scared to reach out but too scared not to. I was stuck in perpetual terror, going down, down, down ...

I'd wake up in a panic, half relieved not to have hit the bottom, as I feared that would come with the news that Derek had died, but scared because there seemed no end to the falling. I couldn't catch my breath. I couldn't stop the terror that at any second Derek would die, that we would all lose him.

Where there is life there is hope. Where there is life there is hope, and hope gets you through everything, I would repeat to myself in my head.

The trouble with hope, though, is that for it to work, you have to believe – you have to have faith that what you hope for is real. Otherwise it is just a wish – a wanting for something absent – for what is not there. If you walk past a gorgeous house and think, I hope I can live in a house like that one day, that 'hope' isn't hope at all: it's a craving. By thinking that way you are encouraging your brain to engage with the fact that you don't live in a house like that. By saying 'one day', you are acknowledging that you are not there now; you are separating yourself from what you want. This sort of longing doesn't give foundation to hope, it does the opposite: it creates an absence, and there is no power in absence. It is a vacuum, a black hole that sucks in any positive energy that could sustain you.

My problem was that even though I had hope that Derek would live, it was constantly being undermined by the fact that the doctors had no cure, and by their warnings that I had to prepare myself as it was likely he would die. So every time I tried to hang on to the best possible outcome I was at the same moment aware of the worst. Fear constantly undermined my hope, and the person I would normally turn to in an emotional crisis was Derek. Only this time he wasn't there.

I wondered what he would advise. I knew that in therapy,

when someone wished for something or had a longing, he would try to break it down into what was behind these longings, what really drove the desire. Why do you want to live in that house? Is it because it would make you feel successful? That you had arrived? Does it remind you of something you craved in your childhood? Is it because you think you would feel safe, secure, have stability? Then he would try to help someone to work through those feelings. What does successful feel like to you? Why does that particular house define success to you? What in your childhood led you to think that way? If you look at a couple and think, I want a love like that, what is it about their behaviour that makes you feel *that* is love? And how could you get those feelings into your life?

But how could I use this knowledge to help me to work through the fear of losing Derek? I knew what I wanted: I wanted him back alive. I wanted our life back. But it was as if for every minute of knowing that he could live I was also grieving his loss and facing the thought of our children losing their father. I was trying to switch grief to hope, but the fear kept flipping it back.

I tried to think how I had coped with crises in the past; after all, I hadn't always had Derek's voice in my ear. I needed a plan. I liked plans: planning for the future usually got me through the pain of 'now'. Dumped by an idiot boyfriend? I knew the drill. I would take to my bed and cry a lot, turn up at friends' houses and drink wine, or go home and indulge in Mum's food while everyone reassured me he wasn't worth it – and I promised myself I'd get fit, look gorgeous, try to win him back or at least show him what he was missing. Any challenge or setback, I could always plan a way out, and I always had friends and family for support.

But how to use any of my usual ruses now? There was no taking to my bed and crying: I had two children looking to me for stability and calm. And lockdown meant I couldn't see anyone. My family were desperate to rush to my aid and take charge so I could focus on Derek. My brother in Cornwall felt cut off: he was desperate to come up to London and give me a hug. For Derek's family it was even worse: not only did they want to support me, they were desperate to be at Derek's bedside too. None of this was possible. Not just for us, of course, but for everyone.

Even though they couldn't physically *be* there to help, they *were* there. Not just my family, the Drapers *and* the Garraways, always at the end of the phone, but friends too. And knowing this – safe in the web of their love and feeling all those good vibrations – gave me strength.

Almost without me knowing, a little team was forming around me. There was my friend Clare Nasir, now a Channel 5 weather presenter, whom I'd met on the first day I joined *GMTV*. There was Vickie White, who had worked in the showbiz department at the same time, and has successfully gone on to other things. And there was Carla Romano, who used to be the LA correspondent for *GMTV*. They formed a WhatsApp group, which worked as a sort of Kate Support Network. And it was brilliant. Carla now lives in New York, so our hours fitted perfectly when I was wired from late-night hospital calls and completely unable to sleep. Clare was there for mystical prayer, sending me links to meditations to help get me to sleep. Vickie was for motivation.

At first I didn't realize that they were in touch with each other, updating one another on what they had discussed or recommended to me. But the network between them also gave them valuable support. They loved Derek too and trying to manage their own feelings as well as support me was taking a huge emotional toll. For example, Vickie has since told me she remembers vividly the moment I told her one particularly bad piece of news. She rang Clare: 'Kate said don't tell anyone but I can't be the only person in the world who knows this.' And Clare now says that every time she walks past the bench she sat on for that conversation she thinks of how her stomach fell through the floor. She is unable to shake the sickening memory.

My friend and *Good Morning Britain* co-presenter Ben Shephard has similar memories: he was getting a tyre replaced on his car, at a particular repair shop, when I called to say that Derek was in hospital, and he has since confessed that it still makes him feel physically sick every time he drives past the place and remembers.

Derek's old friend Ben Wegg-Prosser was always there – by now I spoke to him daily – and even though he was clearly petrified for Derek, he *always* answered the phone with 'What can I do?' It was business-like and efficient, no tears, just instantly ready to help: rushing to get second opinions, find contacts to help us understand Derek's condition better and navigate the flurry of medical opinion. Gloria, too, who had first got us together, had known

Derek most of her adult life and was there on the phone listening and loving.

Each of my close friends reacted to the intensity of emotions in different ways. Some were sympathetic, others practical: 'Do you need milk?' Like Carla, a few were all about motivation: 'Right, get a grip! What are you doing right now? Have you done this? Why not?' Carla would say. And it really helped! She was researching how patients were being treated in the States, then calling me: 'Have you asked them about those? If not, why not?'

Others took care of practicalities I would never have thought of. Tonia Buxton, of the Real Greek restaurants, whom I knew from a cooking strand she had done on *Good Morning Britain*, sent me a text one day: *I'm going to start sending you meals.* I tried to protest, I didn't even know she lived nearby! But she simply said, 'My restaurants are closed. I'm cooking for seven at home anyway so I'm doing it.' And she would turn up on the doorstep, press the buzzer and leave. Those were the days of lockdown when even doing that felt risky, so when I saw the tinfoil platter full of nourishing family food I could have cried with gratitude. All I had to do was to put it in the oven on days when I could hardly feel my own hands.

Then there were Piers Morgan and Susanna Reid, my *Good Morning Britain* colleagues, who were both hugely affected by the situation as they had known Derek well too. Susanna was all about the practical: 'What can I send? What do you need? I'm here if you need to talk, but in the meantime what can I do? Is there something I can send the kids?' And when Piers rang he did what the Piers I've known for twenty years always did, and went into Churchillian rallying mode.

'Right, Kate, get a grip. You're a brilliant journalist. Do what you do best. You know, get on this. Get to the bottom of the situation. You have to fight this. Do not crumble.' He was like a rugby team captain, preparing me for the pitch, quoting every inspirational figure he could from Churchill himself to Nelson Mandela. 'It always seems impossible until it's done.' And it worked, spurring me on.

Very quickly, I realized I had someone for every mood, every time of day, every fresh panic. Just as I started to feel the fear rising in me while I was trying to look after the children, just as I started to lose focus, thinking, Oh my God, I can't go on, they were there, weaving a safety net of love to catch me as I fell.

The senior management at *Good Morning Britain* and Smooth Radio were extraordinarily kind, instantly covering my shifts as I was now in self-isolation and sending me large boxes of food and treats for the kids. Charlotte Hawkins sent a rose bush named 'Hope', Ranvir Singh a fruit basket. More widely across ITV, too, people were so kind. Jeremy Kyle, who had his own troubles at the time, was nothing but generous, eager to help. Others sent messages: the people you wouldn't assume were thinking of you while you were at home digging the garden and trying to cling on to your sanity.

Someone else who came into my life quite randomly, but was a saviour in so many ways, was Rob Rinder, Judge

Rinder from the TV. I had met him many times out and about, and liked him very much. But I don't think I even had his phone number last January. And I certainly didn't know him well enough to call him in a crisis. But one day he texted me saying:

> I've had it. I'm a hypochondriac, I've got absolutely everything drugs-wise that you could need and I've been reading up about it all too. So what can I do?

His straightforwardness made him incredibly easy to deal with, and he was very clear that I could call and ask for whatever I needed, whenever. And he has read almost everything! He never judged me, but tried to help me manage my fears. He approached it like a riddle, a problem-solving challenge to get me to turn my emotions and thoughts to face the right way. He helped me to process things to try to order my thoughts. He would drop everything but never made me feel guilty about it. I knew that his being there was a huge act of friendship, like so many others.

In those days, and weeks, I lived from one second to the next. The only way I could process the feelings and fear was to break time into those tiny chunks. Morning after morning I would wake up and immediately feel gripped by overwhelming terror. It was as if I had been seized by fear. I would lie there, the children often beside me, and try to stabilize myself. I would wait till I felt it was acceptable to call someone, then get up, go downstairs and vent over the phone. Then I'd try to sleep for a bit until the children woke up and I could focus on them. I knew how affected they were by listening to my phone calls, so I tried to get the emotional ones over while they were in bed. Around this time, as I howled down the phone, my mum told me she felt as if she was standing on the other side of a lake watching me drown, unable to save me.

Vickie was living and breathing the sadness with me to the extent that she woke up one night in a cold sweat having dreamt it was her husband Nick who was ill: the terror was so awful she wanted to vomit. Then she saw him sleeping peacefully next to her and felt a huge surge of relief. She started to cry when she thought I must wake up at night and see Derek *not* there and feel the pain without the relief.

It was awful to think of so many people devastated, not just my family but tens of thousands, millions now, of people sick, or fearing the loss of a loved one who was sick, or, worse, in mourning. As a news junkie I've always had news apps on my phone, pinging into my notifications. It used to be exciting. Now the daily pings were numbers of new cases of the virus and a list of the dead. I would feel sick for those whose names I read, and guilty at the surge of relief that Derek's wasn't among them, for that day at least.

One day Rob said to me, 'The only thing I can equate from my life to what you're feeling, and I hope you won't take it as flippant, is that it's like you're waking up every day living minute by minute with the feeling I had on the day I knew I was receiving potentially life-changing exam results. When you wake up and think, Oh my God, my life hinges on this!

At that point it felt as though my entire life, my plans, my dreams for the future rested on one phone call. And whether I had passed or failed. For you, it's whether Derek is alive or dead. I can remember that feeling as unbearable. I don't know how you're coping with it so endlessly.' It dawned on me as he said this that it was because of people like him that I could cope. That like thousands of others up and down the country, I was finding a way to keep going and hoping for the best by drawing on the support of friends.

By now I was getting messages from all sorts of stars of stage and screen, genuine personal notes of comfort, offering help. David Beckham messaged me on Instagram. I hadn't had the chance to look at social media so it was Darcey and Billy who spotted it (always much more plugged in than I am) and squealed with delight. I messaged him back, thanking him and saying the kids were thrilled. He sent a personal video to each of them, words of encouragement and fun. It was wonderful to see them smiling. He said he had been thinking of his own kids and how they might feel, which was so kind of him.

Then Sir Elton John called. Yes, *the* Sir Elton John. I was blowing up the paddling pool at the time, trying to distract the kids with water fun, in those unseasonably blistering spring days. When the phone rang I ran to it in case it was the hospital.

'Hi,' he said, 'it's Elton here. I'm so sorry I haven't called before.'

I had met him for interviews over the years, when he was always great fun and friendly. But this was different, him not answering questions but offering to help. He had a friend who had been seriously ill in a coma for two weeks in early February and he wanted to know what drugs the doctors here in the UK had tried on Derek. His pioneering work with his AIDS foundation meant that he knew a lot of doctors who were expert in antiviral medicine, which was being trialled for use against Covid in the US. I realized he was calling from Los Angeles, and that he genuinely meant it when he said he wanted to do something – and even more that he might actually be able to make a difference. Before long I was taking notes, not thinking of him as Elton the star whose music I loved and could easily have been playing on my iPhone right then, but as someone who was reaching out as a friend. In the end it was too late for Derek: the virus had progressed too far for antivirals to have any impact. But later on I needed help from Elton and he came through yet again.

People from all sides of the political fence wanted to know if they could help. Tony Blair called, so worried for Derek, saying he would pass on any medical developments he heard of from across the world. The prime minister, Boris Johnson, wrote me the most tender personal note about Derek, recalling fun times they'd had when he worked at the *Spectator*. It was a frightening time for him and for his fiancée, Carrie, especially as she was expecting her first baby. So they had more reason than most to empathize. These weren't political manoeuvres but human gestures. I felt like I was seeing the best of people in the worst of times.

Lord Mandelson wrote to Derek's mother. He had worked

with Derek for years and he said some wonderful things about the good Derek had done and the kind of person he is. I know it lifted her hugely: she needed to hear that he was loved and respected, that his life had purpose just when it was at its greatest risk of being snatched away.

It was so heartening to feel Derek was appreciated, uplifting and sustaining. Hundreds of thousands of people were now messaging me on Instagram too. Some were just sending love, or sharing stories of loss and how they had got through it. Others were writing with tales of miraculous recoveries from injuries and disease that they wanted me to take heart from. All of them were saying, 'Never give up hope. Never give up hope.' I would read those messages at night when I couldn't sleep, nourished by how much energy and thought had gone into sending them.

'It's so wonderful,' I told Rob one day, 'but I feel guilty. There are so many people up and down the country going through this and they might not have this outpouring of love. They might be going through it alone.'

'But they might not be, Kate,' he said. 'They will have their own family, friends, and their own community. This is what people *do*. Our humanity is our best quality.'

'I suppose so ...'

'Whatever you put out into the universe will come back to you,' he told me. 'For twenty years you have got up at dawn and been bright and breezy, and people have related to you. And they're now sending back that positive energy to you because people *are* good.

'Look,' he persisted. 'You've told me that you used to say

when you went on air that "No matter how bad your day's been, there will always be someone watching who's had a worse day and it's your job to make them smile." You said it gave your work extra purpose beyond being a journalist to try to put them in a better mood, to deal with whatever was on their mind that day. *You* put that energy out there, so accept it now that it's coming back to you.'

I wasn't convinced it was any of my doing but I could see that people were good. Maybe this was the way we were going to get through this: with love. *That* was the way hope could be made real.

One day I received a letter from the office of a member of the Royal Family. How lovely, I thought, although it seemed utterly surreal. I was living through the worst days my life could ever hold and the Royal Family were delivering letters to my front door.

It turned out they wanted to offer the services of a royal physician. A day or two later, I received a call from the doctor, who turned out to be very senior at another London hospital and was interested in Derek's case. He asked to see Derek's CT scans, and talked to his doctors about his condition. He then called back and said he was having great care, but it was just a case of 'wait and see'. He said, 'Kate, the truth is, it's only great care that will save him now. We have people who come in and they don't make it, and we have people who come in looking like they're done for but they recover. We're treating them all the same. At the moment, we're fighting an enemy we just don't understand.'

How incredible to have been so thought-of. It was as if life had come to such a standstill globally that anyone with a heart was trying to do something practical to help. Every time events seemed to show that there was no hope for Derek, suddenly, from somewhere completely unexpected, hope came. From the love in the world.

This sense of us all being in it together, that we were all connected, felt very intense at this point in that first lockdown. It wasn't just celebrities doing their thing: I took huge solace from the actions of neighbours and people I had barely spoken to before. Even though it was painful for me to go out to Clap for Carers, I felt very strongly that I needed to see people laughing and joking. I felt as if I was part of something so special because we were so directly affected by those very carers. People were crossing the road to check on elderly neighbours who were shielding, knowing they probably hadn't seen anyone all week.

The rest of the week, neighbours would call or leave notes or even shout over the fence, letting me know when they were running errands for people who were ill or older so couldn't go out. I will never forget the overwhelming warmth and gratitude we felt when someone passed our house and dropped off a lemon drizzle cake.

Hope seemed to spring up in the most unexpected places, from the PE instructors leading whole streets in outdoor exercise classes, to the teacher who built a fairy grotto at the end of her garden to cheer up bored and lonely children, to the woman who lived across the road from me. One morning she crossed the street, which was as far as any of us dared to go in those first few months of learning the art of social distancing.

'Hi, you've lived over the road from me for years and we've only ever really nodded hello. But eleven years ago my husband had a car crash and was in a coma for a long time. Let me help you with this.' I could hardly believe it. This quiet woman, whose life I had never imagined, must have felt such pain. But there she was, giving me a handful of pointers on how to cope.

First, she told me that the whole situation was going to be really tough on me. 'But you have to eat,' she said. 'And you have to eat really good food. You also need to know that you're not going to be able to manage this perfectly. You have to let go of that.'

OK ... I nodded, reeling slightly.

'But there *is* hope. I was told that my husband would be permanently brain-damaged. He had a car accident where he was knocked off his bicycle and was told he would never walk again, might never come out of the coma. And it took a long time, but he did. He's walking. He's talking. He's back. But it was a *looong* time.'

I was floored, because this was someone who had been in a comparable situation, and she was saying concrete things rather than just woolly suggestions to 'Think positive'. It may sound harsh, but when someone says, 'Think positive,' with nothing to back it up, it's so hard to do. You're surrounded by evidence of the negative, so you need evidence *for* hope. If you have none, talk of positivity can wound you more. You just think, But that's not going to be me!

Those around me, and those from unexpected quarters, were offering me hope, when the facts of my situation seemed only to offer negativity.

It wasn't just my own circumstances that were so troubling either. It was at this point that the prime minister, Boris Johnson, became ill with the disease. While doctors started to admit they weren't sure about the path of the coronavirus, and scientists started to admit they did not have all of the data we needed, and parents admitted they had no idea how to home school and hold down jobs at the same time, our leader himself proved just as fallible. Days after reassuring us that he was fine, working away at home, he appeared looking worryingly ill. And days after that, only hours after Downing Street had told us he was doing well, he was admitted to hospital.

The pillars that had been supporting normal life suddenly seemed as if they might not be up to the job. The people we had all relied on to have the answers, to be in control of things, were revealing themselves to be just as flawed as I had always felt – as we had all felt. Yes, there was something reassuring about this, knowing that we were all of us struggling during these strange days. But there was also something terrifying: who was in charge? Who *was* up to the job? Who knew how to get any of us, from Derek to the nation as a whole, out of this? As a journalist I had a career, a life, spent searching for the facts, looking at how to get to the essence of a story. But when I looked at this story, it seemed to warp and fade whenever I tried to grasp a truth, a certainty, anything that might prove to be solid. And, as with my situation, the nation had to do the same: we waited. We hoped that things would improve. We hoped that the news would change. We hoped that we would make it, but mostly we all did the same thing. We waited.

What we were going through felt global. But while it was a horrific time, it was also a time in which, when all seemed so bleak, certainty came from the evidence of good in people, and the power of positive energy. If anything was going to get me, any of us, through it was that. But first I had to work out how the children and I were going to get through each day.

Chapter 6

Fear

At some point since the pandemic took over our lives I think we've all been assailed by fear: fear of getting ill, fear for our loved ones, fear for our livelihoods, or the fear that grips you when you feel lonely, cut off, or when all that you hold dear is in jeopardy.

I was realizing that simply living minute by minute in this state wasn't sustainable for me or for the children. I had to be there for them – *really* there for them – and for Derek. I was simply trying to spin too many plates not very well. I had somehow to find a way to manage my time and, most importantly, a fear that wasn't going to go away.

Whenever we planned anything as a family, Derek would always get out a pen, paper and a pack of highlighter pens. In 2007, when I was grappling with the decision of whether to do *Strictly Come Dancing*, he did just that. I really wanted to be part of such an incredible show but Darcey was just sixteen months old, and I was working every day on *GMTV*. I knew from friends who had taken part in it that the amount of training required was huge, and that the show inevitably took over your life. So, Derek carved up my day on paper for me: red represented time with Darcey, blue was for *GMTV*, and pink was for *Strictly* training. It was only after we had chopped up our time and worked out how Derek could manage his work so that he could spend more time at home with Darcey that he said, 'Oh, no! I haven't got a colour for you and me! Never mind, we have all the time in the world.'

I prayed that we still did.

I didn't get out the highlighter pens this time but I knew I had ruthlessly to block things off in some way, manage one project at a time and really be involved in each one. One day Susanna Reid sent a box of Lego for Billy and Darcey. Her boys had got really into it during lockdown and she thought my two would like it too. The picture on the box showed that it was huge – more than two thousand pieces. It was two buildings, a petrol pump and a bookshop, all of it tall and incredibly detailed.

'Oh, wow! I can use my Lego characters too! Darcey, we can create a whole town!' Billy was thrilled. 'Can we do it now?'

Two pairs of eyes looked at me almost nervously, as if their owners thought they were about to be disappointed.

'Maybe Mum has things to do, Bill,' Darcey said. 'You know, with Dad.'

I looked at their little faces. They were children. This was

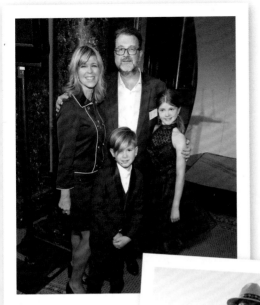

Left: At the launch for Derek's book, *Create Space*. Darcey said we should all wear dark blue, the colour of his company CDP's branding.

Right: The trip of a lifetime! Derek hired an RV to take us across California to revisit places he loved when he was studying at Berkeley.

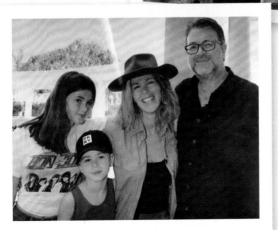

Left: Post-jungle and excited about the year ahead.

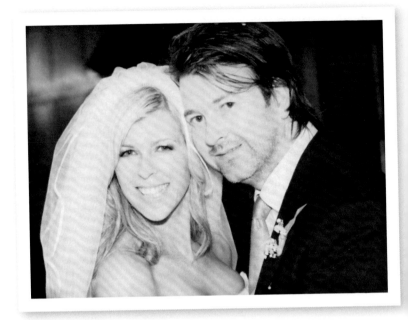

Our wedding day.

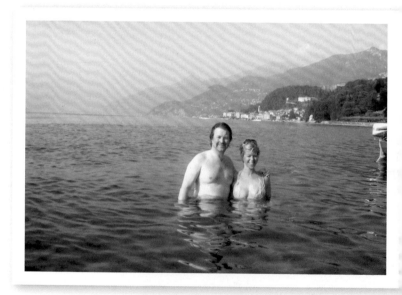

'That picture' of us on holiday in Lake Como which Derek
keeps in his Thinking Room.

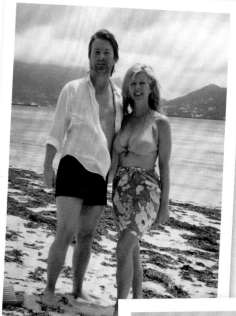

Left: The last holiday we had as a couple before the children arrived and changed everything. Derek wanted us to celebrate each other as we strolled along Caribbean beaches. I was seven months pregnant with swollen ankles but it still felt romantic.

Right: The photo of Derek, Darcey and me that Derek keeps in his office.

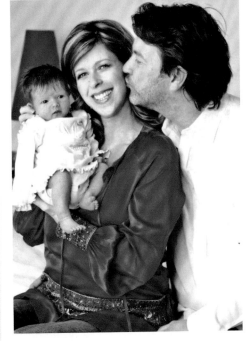

Right: Derek loves this photo of him with Darcey because it is typical of their relationship from the start: total adoration from him; Darcey less than impressed!

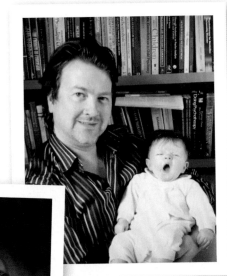

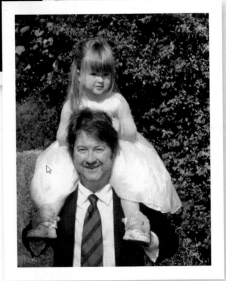

Left: Derek showing off Billy at the church where we had our first date – St Mary's, Primrose Hill.

Right: Derek the carriage to Darcey's bridesmaid.

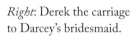

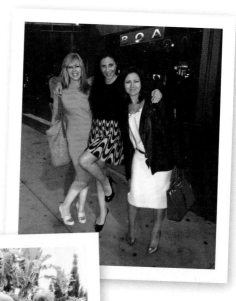

Right: Partying in LA with Carla (*centre*) and Gloria, who introduced Derek and me. We left our husbands at home!

Left: On holiday with Gloria (in yellow), her husband James (*centre*), Clare and her husband Chris Hawkins. Derek is taking the photo.

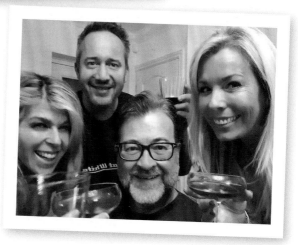

Right: Celebrating 'White Christmas' with Vickie and Nick White.

Right: Derek's photograph of Boxing Day 2019. Clockwise from the left: me, my brother Matthew, Billy, my dad and mum, Darcey, my niece Jen and my sister-in-law Geri.

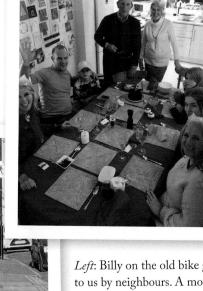

Left: Billy on the old bike given to us by neighbours. A moment of joy.

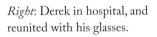

Right: Derek in hospital, and reunited with his glasses.

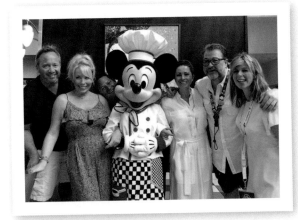

Right: Amazing friends and my support system. Here we are with Vickie and Nick, Clare and Chris, on holiday in Disneyland.

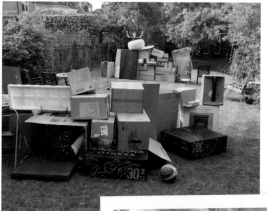

Left: The box forts and gym blocks.

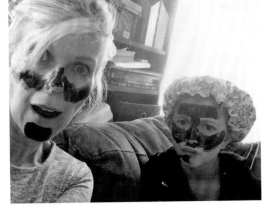

Right: Darcey's Day Spa: getting ready for the return to GMB – face masks, leg wax and even a hair trim from her.

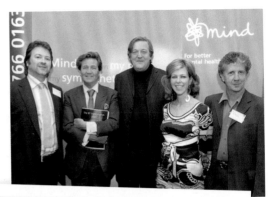

Right: One of Derek's proudest moments: Winner of Mind Mental Health Journalist of the Year, 2009.

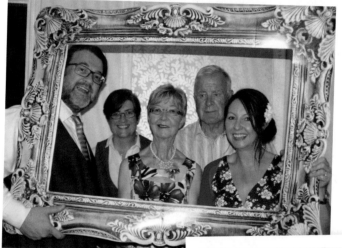

Above: Derek and his sisters, Di (left) and Sue with their parents at Chrina and Ken's golden wedding anniversary.

Right: Who does he think he is?! My hero.

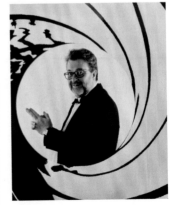

their childhood. Another day passing for me was another day that Derek had lived, another day to hope that things might get better. For them, it was another day of their childhood spent waiting, fearfully wondering. Since the day Derek had got into the ambulance, saying he would be back soon, the nightmare had gone on unfathomably long for them. Days when they feared their beloved daddy was in peril. They didn't know the detail, of course, but they knew what Covid was, that Dad had it and that people died from it. They could hear my fear on the phone and I'm sure they picked up scraps of information, however much I tried to squirrel myself away to make calls.

They had had weeks of this, days when they were struggling to wrestle childhood joy out of all of this fear. I was conflicted by this. Every time they did something cute or comical, something so *them*, my heart would leap, and I would imagine Derek laughing. A friend who has two boys and whose husband had died a few years before had once said to me that it's the loneliest feeling on earth when you see your kids do something you know only their dad would truly appreciate. No one else takes pleasure in the same way from the things they do or say. Friends can be proud, grandparents dote, but it was only with her husband that my friend felt that deep connection of stomach-aching love and joy they both shared. I now know exactly what she meant. These days, I would look at our kids and feel a surge of joy, then, almost in the next breath, the fear.

What if Derek never gets to have this again? What if he never sees them grow up, to flourish, to bloom, to become the wonderful human beings he believed they were going to be? And what if they lost him? Their rock, their guru, their playmate, their adviser – their dad?

It was unbearable. The fear slashed through the joy. But they *needed* their joy, and they needed it even more now. I pushed the fears down with one thought, a steel boot kicking anything else away: I had to experience that joy with them as fully as I could *because* Derek couldn't do so right now. I had to experience it with them *for* him.

'Yes, we can!' I said. 'I'm going to put the phone over here just so that if the hospital calls we don't miss it, and then I'm all yours.'

They squealed (well, Darcey did so as much as any teenager squeals) as we tumbled the Lego pieces out on to the floor and studied the instructions, losing ourselves in its colourful brick world, where instructions were reliable and walls became solid in an instant. Even Darcey, usually less of a Lego fan than Bill, joined in with gusto. We were soon rowing over who had put a wrong piece where, laughing as I got the instructions muddled and generally experiencing an enormous, blissful dollop of normality. In fact, it was so normal that I sent a video of them putting the last piece on top of the first building to Susanna. She was thrilled for us, as it had given us exactly what she had hoped for.

When the hospital rang, wrenching me back to the gut-churning anxiety of the present, the children were happy to continue with the world-building on their own.

'Don't worry, Mum, I'm going to do some stop-motion animation,' Bill said (he has an app on his iPad for this).

'We'll show you after,' he called, as I scrambled out of the door to speak away from their ears.

That was how we inched our way forward through this time, snatching joy where we could. The blissful April sunshine and the fact we were lucky enough to have a garden helped too. We were living to our own crazy timetable. Late-night calls disrupted any normal bedtime, which meant the children were sleeping late. So, when I came off a call after midnight one night, and Darcey said, 'Can we all go in the paddling pool … now?' I thought, Why not? The gleam in her eye, the sheer rebellious nature of it all was pure joy. Then, when it finally got too cold, we sprinted inside to a hot bath and cuddled up in bed with the fan heater on full blast, exhausted in all the right ways, cosy and safe.

On the nights when it was too chilly for the paddling pool, our battered old trampoline came into play. We had been meaning to get a new one for ages, but then Derek had got sick and I couldn't find one as they had sold out everywhere. Everyone seemed to have decided that if they were stuck in their gardens, they might as well make it as fun as possible.

But it worked. We flung ourselves around like lunatics, the kids with skill and terrifying height, me with enthusiasm and comedy. Then, when we were all exhausted, we took to sitting on the trampoline and chatting. One night, Darcey dragged a huge dust sheet out of our basement and stretched it over the top. She had seen a video on YouTube called 'trampoline camping'. We sat under it and chatted for hours, Bill calling it 'our daily dose of gossip'. Not that we really had any gossip – no one was going anywhere. But we played 'Would you rather?' and other games. They teased each other about who they thought they fancied at school, we talked about grandparents, cousins and friends, the people they were missing so much. And we talked about it in that kiddish way: 'I wonder what Lucy will be when she grows up'; 'Do you think Eddie is walking now?'; 'What shall we get Eleanor for her first birthday?'; 'Granddad would hate that. His favourite thing to do is …' It brought those precious people back into our lives, making them feel real when they couldn't be there. They talked about Derek, too, but not about him being sick: about him being alive.

'Do you remember when Dad wore that ridiculous hat?'

'When he jumped in the pool on holiday and soaked that lady?'

And so on. They were keeping him alive in all our minds, bringing him here with us in the garden, trying in their own way to fill the absence they so keenly felt.

Heaven knows what the neighbours thought of us, squealing and splashing around until all hours, but I noticed they were often up early, playing in their own gardens, presumably before they had to start working and home schooling. It was lovely to hear, everyone trying to find pockets of joy and love while they juggled the challenge of lockdown. In a way it was liberating to be set free from the shackles of normal timetables, to be able to enjoy the gardens that had been out of bounds during the daily nine-to-five for years.

The garden became our sanctuary through those aching weeks of waiting. I could sit outside on the phone watching them play, shouting an occasional 'Well done!' or 'Be careful!' and join in with them as soon as the call was over.

We had bought the house because of the garden. I loved gardening, but, until this house, I had never had my own, and neither had Derek. The house he grew up in had had a flagged backyard and after that he had lived in flats. When we moved in, the garden was wild and overgrown, but we had loved its wildness – it had felt like an escape from the city. Eventually we had to sort it out, but as we hacked things back Derek begged me to keep some signature plants (or rather weeds!), things we remembered from when we had first moved in. We'd needed to clear a space for the kids to play as the patch that could barely have been called a lawn was covered with brambles. But Derek didn't want them completely gone. 'Wait!' he had said. 'Just keep one bush, you know, for the memories and for the blackberries in autumn!'

There were wild irises too, huge ones, which flowered briefly before withering to pretty uninteresting reeds. They were everywhere, their huge tubers creeping around, connecting underground, preventing me from planting anything more interesting. But Derek loved them – they were as precious to him as any award-winning rose. Suddenly I was desperate for them to thrive. I tended them that summer as though I was entering a flower show: fertilizing, watering, watching. It didn't take a psychologist as qualified as Derek to know that keeping those flowers going was, on some level, about trying to keep Derek going too.

Sometimes, in the early hours of the morning, when I

woke up clammy with fear, I would creep out of bed, trying not to wake the children, make myself a cup of tea and sit in the garden, watching the reeds moving in the night breeze. It was beautiful, mesmeric. Calming.

I guess those moments were me practising a kind of mindfulness. As I understand it, mindfulness meditation means sitting silently and paying attention to your thoughts, your breath and your body. Rather than saying to yourself, 'No! Stop thinking about that stressful thing!' or trying to work out how to overcome the stress, just sit and acknowledge that sometimes things *are* really stressful, that it's not wrong to feel that way. Just sitting in the garden, not trying to *force* myself to sleep because I *had* to sleep, but acknowledging that I needed to sit, in peace, for a while, felt like my version of mindfulness.

A friend of mine who is a psychologist (one of the support network that was forming around me) told me I needed to start doing this more. He explained to me that the state of simply sitting and *being* (rather than endlessly solving, communicating, learning, panicking) was not wishy-washy hippie nonsense, but that it had medical science behind it. Great! I thought. A fact! I loved a fact: it was steadying.

He explained that the medulla – the part of our brain stem that controls stress hormones – is designed to release adrenalin, the fight-or-flight hormone, in moments of crisis. It is there to help us stay awake when a predator might be close, run from an encroaching avalanche, or lift the boulder that might trap our frightened child. It's a hugely powerful hormone that is meant to help us *in emergencies*.

But sloshing endless adrenalin into our systems can be damaging in the long term. The very fact that it is so powerful in the short term is what can make it almost toxic in the long term: I was at risk of letting the constant state of peril make me ill as well.

'You need to pick something, and totally focus on that one thing. Push everything else out of your mind for a bit,' he explained. 'It helps if it's something that stimulates the senses.'

I remembered my time in the jungle: we were starved of flavours other than rice and beans, so when we were given something different to eat we were euphoric about it. One time we were given a segment of orange. It was so delicious – so bright, so *orange*! – that we ate slowly, smelling the flesh first, sucking the juice, feeling the texture on our tongues. It made me realize how much we take food for granted, eating while we watch TV, barely tasting it at all. As this thought popped into my head, I went to the fruit bowl, got an orange and focused on it hard as I ate every mouthful. That was something I began doing more and more when things overwhelmed me.

Not long after this, my friend Vickie said that now I had mindfulness in my arsenal, it was time to try manifesting. She believed in it, and was keen for me to try.

'Write down everything you want,' she explained. 'And don't hold back!'

'I just want him to live,' I replied forlornly.

'No, you must be specific. You want detail. You really want to be able to imagine it. What do you want to do together when he gets well?' (Note she said when not if; it doesn't work if you allow doubt to creep in.) 'Put detail in: What you will eat. What he will be wearing. Where you will go. Build a picture and colour it in as much as possible with detail. Writing these things down is what makes it concrete, a manifestation, not just a wish,' Vickie explained. 'It's all positive.'

So I wrote down everything that I wanted to do with Derek: every café I wanted to visit with him, every meal I wanted us to share, every walk I wanted us to go on. I wrote specific descriptions of him, in his chair in the garden, enjoying his irises in full bloom, just as I was sure he longed to be doing.

And those manifestations are still under my pillow to this day.

Sometimes, when I wanted to feel close to Derek, I would head up to the attic to his Thinking Room, with his Buddhas, his candles, his crucifix, and the little bits and pieces that helped him when he was stressed or sad, and I'd try to think of him. I had taken other pictures of him up to that room. I would stare into his eyes and tell him to stay with me, and pray to God to save him. I knew Derek was religious and, even though I didn't go to church every Sunday, as he did, I believe in God. So I prayed with all my might, always saying, 'I may not be worthy but *he* believes in you, save *him*.'

By now friends were giving me prayers, specific ones that I repeated every day: prayers to saints, Carla suggesting Papa Pio, and prayers to Buddhist monks, Clare Nasir saying, 'Babba Gee, save Derek.'

There was a power in the words, their positive energy. The process of focusing and trying to connect with an energy beyond man's reason was transporting. After all, every religion passed down through the centuries has a form of prayer included in its ritual so there must be some purpose, some usefulness to it.

Whether you believe prayer can heal is a different matter, but I knew Derek understood prayer to be a strong nourishing force for those who trusted in it. In his as yet unpublished book *The Psychology of Everyday Life* he writes about how often he is struck by how many in long-term therapy eventually come to explore spirituality, even if they don't classify themselves as religious. He writes that the urge 'to connect with something more mystical and beyond themselves seems always to coincide with real progress in treatment'.

This book was due to be published when he had fallen ill, and one of the last things he did was send a copy of the manuscript to Susanna Reid for her comments. Susanna picked this up again when she was thinking about Derek's plight and found herself rereading this chapter. One section looked at studies conducted into the effects of prayer on the body.

'Studies show that people who pray or meditate have lower blood pressure, stress levels and incidence of depression. Still more studies claim to prove that having someone pray for you, even if you aren't aware of it, can lead to better recovery from heart disease and breast cancer.'

Susanna really isn't a prayer person, but she messaged me to say that Derek explained prayer, and what it meant in terms of energy, so meticulously that she 'got it' in a way she never had before and within seconds she had put the book down and said a prayer for Derek.

I don't know if you can prove prayer works, but I think we all have the proof of our own eyes that energy has an impact, positive and negative. We see it when someone has positive energy: good things happen. Conversely those who focus on the negative always seem to find it.

And, anyway, what harm could it do when science could give me no concrete answers, when doctors all around the world were being left with a lot of 'I don't know'? This was all trickling down to every patient, every family affected by Covid.

Every time I spoke to the doctors they tried to ready me for the worst news. I was constantly hearing from them, 'He might die, he might die, he might die,' and it was inevitably drawing me into a negative energy. I genuinely believe that. On a practical level, I understood why they had to do it, but I needed something to counteract the emotional impact, and all of those techniques were helping me to stay positive.

Lizzie Cundy was sending me, via a friend, recordings of American preachers saying, 'HEAL DEREK NOW!' which I asked the nurses to play to him as he lay there. There were days when the kids and I were almost hysterical with laughter because it was so loud and *so* American.

But who knows? It might have worked. It might have drifted through to him, and how cheering would it have been for Derek to know that this force of goodwill was spurring him on? Other friends sent me details of mystics and healers who had helped them in the past. They believed in them and it helped to get a text from them oozing confidence that I had reason to hope. It gave me strength to keep going.

Linda Lusardi, after hearing about Derek, reached out to me out of the blue. She wanted to see if she could help as she had been seriously ill in hospital, fearing she was going to die as a result of Covid. Her husband was good friends with June Field, a spiritual healer, and he asked June to send Linda some remote healing. Linda was unaware of this but immediately afterwards she felt a wave of positivity. She rang her husband and said, 'I am going to get better.' That was as concrete as anything else I had heard that day so why not? I got her involved immediately. None of these healers was charging a penny: they just wanted to help. That in itself was a wonderful thing, that goodness, to bring into Derek's life.

'Why not?' This was what I asked myself time and again, as I had to make a huge shift, opening myself to all sorts of new ideas. I had to put aside the life I'd always known, which had been built on facts. After all, the basis of every journalistic report and every interview I did was 'get your facts straight'. And suddenly there were no facts. Only people, from medical specialists to government, saying, 'We don't know, we don't know, we don't know.'

In a universe where you have no facts to cling to, when the biggest brains in the world are saying, 'There is no data,' you have to change how you see the world, and say to yourself, 'Hang on, I am surrounded by incredible love.' From people on Twitter, Instagram, Facebook, close friends, neighbours, celebrities I barely knew: all sorts of people were messaging me and saying, 'My husband/son/grandfather is in hospital too. I feel your pain. I am sending you love.' And I tried to send it right back, to keep the energy going.

I felt that in the life he had led and the work he had done, Derek was now moving people to help, to pray for him when he needed it. So many of his friends were leaving messages for me to play to him down the phone while he lay in hospital. I could listen to those messages while I was playing them to him, about moments they had had together, things he had done for them that I didn't even know about. His former therapy clients, people he had worked with in politics, all sorts. It was as if it was keeping Derek alive in a spiritual sense as well as a literal one. It made me feel his energy had gone out into the world and now those people he had interacted with were keeping that energy afloat. And I know it was keeping me going.

Meanwhile, my conventional research continued. I was in touch with research projects all over the world who were looking into repurposing techniques used to treat other conditions, exploring how they might be used to tackle Covid and its effects. I was talking to scientists in Australia who were trying out how stem-cell drugs and techniques might help if used early enough in the infection.

Individual researchers were contacting me, asking about Derek and his treatments so far, wondering if they might be able to do something positive. But I was told Derek was too weak to try anything new. Constantly, the refrain was 'Wait and see. He is hanging by a thread.' It also turned out that we were so often just too late for a treatment to be worth trying. Everyone was trying so hard, but at every turn it seemed we were playing catch-up.

I had tried everything I could to research, to persuade, to advocate. I had used all the skills I had in my public life, searching for facts and tugging at leads. And I had used all of my personal skills, trying to keep home life afloat, trying to stay focused on hope for all of us. Now, the best use of my time during this endless waiting seemed to be talking to Derek, turning what felt like a passive process on its head, into active waiting.

There were two points in the day when I could do it. Late in the evening when the staff were arriving for the night shift, a nurse could hold the phone to his ear, allowing me to talk directly to Derek from home. When the morning shift appeared, I would speak to the phone resting by his ear. These turned into intense, private times when I could focus on Derek mentally. I would try to banish thoughts of treatment, or outcomes, or life beyond him and me, and find a place where I could connect with him.

But it went beyond that. I wanted him to know that if he was somewhere far away, fighting an internal battle, the kids and I were still here, waiting for him, thinking about him, planning for him. I would chat into the phone for as long as I could, telling him about holidays we were going to have together, things we would do with the children, things we would do to the house, and beyond. We didn't know if he could hear, but I could imagine how lonely he would feel if he could hear and *not* know that we were all rooting for him.

I was also trying to make sure that what he could hear was more positive, more calming than it had been during those first few chaotic days after he was admitted. It must have been so terrifying to hear the mayhem, shouting and raw pain all around him and have no voice of his own. Now, I wondered if the silence on the ward might be frightening. He was surrounded by people in comas, so while it was calmer, the ominous and often indecipherable beeps and bleeps of medical equipment formed the only sonic landscape. If he could hear, would he even have a sense of where he was? Just in case, I would whisper to him daily:

'You're somewhere safe. You're being looked after. I'm in touch with everyone. I've been talking to your father this morning, and I had a good chat with your friend Ben after that …'

Anything I could think of to say that would encourage him to survive, to come back to us, to leave the dark space he must have been in, I would say it.

You have to come back, you have to hear about the good you've done.

I know you're in there, Derek, I know you're there.

I would also whisper these things to him as I sat in the Thinking Room, and I carried the thoughts with me through the weeks as we waited to know if Derek had lived for another minute, another hour, another day.

I had nothing to measure progress by but eventually the hospital assigned one person, Dr C, to update me daily. I asked him if he felt he had drawn a short straw. He laughed.

'Well, you do ask a *lot* of questions but there's nothing wrong with that!' He chuckled. 'To be honest, most families just call and want to know if their loved one is OK, but I'll brief you on the urgent questions from now on.'

It was a relief. He got me, explained everything to me in detail – he was a lifeline. He had hope: he understood its power.

'You know,' he told me one day, 'we doctors don't say it enough but we *are* getting survivors. As time goes on we are learning more and more, so hang in there, Kate.'

I took that nugget of hope, and thought back to how I had started off in late March, when I had used 'Why him?' and 'Why not him?' to still my sense of unfairness. Now, I realized, I could think, 'Why not him?' about survival, rather than the illness: he might be one of the *lucky* ones. After all, I told myself, trying to harness as much of that positive energy as possible, why *shouldn't* he be one of the survivors? *Why not him?*

As time ticked by, Dr C helped me to manage how I digested the daily updates. He was someone to measure the days with, little steps forwards, better oxygen levels today and so on. He taught me to try to look at lots of different measurements over two or three days and not to panic or jump with glee if there was a slight fluctuation. And there was one thing he was sure about.

'It's all about the lungs, Kate. We have to get his lungs moving. And we have to get him off ECMO. But, for now, it's all about the lungs. I would just keep going …'

So we did. We just kept going. By late spring things

slowly started to shift. Boris Johnson was discharged from intensive care, then from hospital, and at last, I had some good news too. This state of active waiting, something less than helping but more than patience, eventually seemed to bear fruit when one day towards the end of April Dr C rang up and said that Derek's oxygen and infection levels had reached a point where they could start to wean him off the ECMO machine. The process is very delicate, not a simple on-and-off switch. He needed to have the amount of oxygen in the flow of blood going into the machine gradually reduced, until they could be confident his lungs were working well enough to keep him alive. He would still need to be on a ventilator and was a long way from breathing on his own but this was a start. It was a slow, anxious process. They would reduce the flow for a day or two, then the oxygen levels in his blood would drop too much, meaning the ventilator alone still wasn't enough, so the flow had to be increased again. All the while, there was a risk to his heart, and, of course, he was still on kidney dialysis and liver support. Derek was still in a highly critical condition.

Slowly, patiently, delicately, they continued. And then one morning Dr C called me. 'We've done it. He's off ECMO. He's been off, and on his own, for twenty-four hours actually but we didn't want to tell you in case it had to go back up again. But he's free and the tubes are out.'

'Oh, that's amazing!' It was the week before my birthday and the sun was out. Maybe things really were turning around.

'Look, we're not out of the woods yet,' he continued. 'We

have to stabilize him long term, and we don't want to move him from this ward for a little while, just in case. What we have to do next is to reduce the paralysis drugs and the sedation he has been on. In short, we have to wake him up. But, so far, this is good progress.'

Another agonizingly slow process, but one suffused with positivity. They reduced the drugs, bit by bit, hoping that as they left his system he would come round, open his eyes and be back to us. I started to visualize the scenes I had seen on the news: long-term Covid patients being clapped as they left the ward, waving at the teams who had cared for them as they were wheeled away, smiling. Instead, every time Derek's doctors decreased his sedation, his heart rate would shoot up so they had to take him deeper into the coma again. They were constantly tweaking, balancing kidneys, lungs, heart, liver, trying to work out how they could gently, effectively rouse him from his coma.

During this process, which should normally take about seventy-two hours, Derek displayed behaviours that seemed to confuse the medical team. He opened his eyes, but his stare was blank. He was just unresponsive, they would say. Then there would be good news: he was 'tracking', following noise or movement around a room, a little like a newborn baby does. He might not necessarily be alert and watching, but aware, trying to trace where noise or movement was happening. The team thought he might be able to hear, but they still weren't sure.

Then one day he wiggled his toes. But in the days that followed, nothing. Had that first movement been involuntary?

Or had he felt a genuine sensation? They didn't know. How could they? It was all unknown. Few people they had treated with Covid had been in a coma for so long and certainly none as badly affected as Derek. At one point he started to jerk, almost as if he was fitting. Was this him coming round, or a sign of more problems?

This went on for a couple of weeks. One day it would seem he was rousing, but the next he would be back in the unresponsive state. Eventually a member of the intensive-care team said to me that she thought he was 'pickled'. I had no idea what she meant, until she explained that sometimes patients live under sedation for so long that it takes longer for them to come round.

What was complicating everything was the unknown damage that Covid caused the body to do to itself with its extreme immune response. We were all learning that the problem was twofold: the damage the disease had done, and the damage that the body had done to itself while fighting, inflamed, raging with every resource it had.

Perhaps this slow rousing was simply part of that, the team wondered. Because Covid is, in essence, inflammation. It causes inflammation. Initially, when people were first getting sick it was seen as primarily a lung disease because those who were dying had acute respiratory failure. Now they were learning that Covid attacks every organ in the body; every cell could be affected, damaged, destroyed by Covid inflammation. This is part of the reason why we are seeing more and more cases of Long Covid: people who weren't particularly sick with the virus, which hadn't much affected their lungs, were discovering that other organs in the body had been affected, long after their supposed recovery. Hospitals were reporting an increase in encephalitis, inflammation of the brain, in people who later tested positive for Covid: when they arrived in hospital they had had no cough or temperature so no one connected the two. They had come into hospital complaining of dizziness, sickness and nausea. Slowly the teams working around the world realized that Covid had led to encephalitis. So was this what was going on?

As anxiety-provoking as these suggestions were, there were still huge gains. The day Derek was strong enough to be given a tracheotomy, an incision in his windpipe, to breathe through marked a huge milestone. Weeks before, Dr C had said, 'When they tell you he is well enough to have a tracheotomy, now *that* is a day to celebrate.' Because it would mean that he was strong enough to survive the procedure. I will never forget the glow of hope I felt the day that Dr C rang saying that the procedure had gone ahead. He was delighted, but as cautious as specialists always are. 'I wouldn't open the champagne yet,' he told me, 'but I think you can put a bottle in the fridge ...'

At this point, because of how ill he had been and how severe the lockdown restrictions were at that time, I had not laid eyes on him, in real life or online, for weeks. So the day they suggested getting in an iPad for me to talk to him was a huge shock. The team was standing around his bed talking, when suddenly I saw Derek there.

Once I had gathered myself enough to look properly, I

searched the gaze I had known so well for so long: I had seen Derek with so many expressions, love, laughter, fury, but I had never looked into his eyes and seen a stare so blank.

During the past few weeks I had built a great relationship with the team looking after him. We understood each other. They trusted that I was never questioning things because I was challenging their work: they knew that for me it was just about knowing, understanding and trying to be as useful as possible. I understood that they really were trying everything they could with the resources and research they had. Now I had the impression that they were no longer keen to let on how worried they might be but I could tell they were increasingly concerned as to why he wasn't responding. It seemed they feared it was less and less likely to be just an effect of the coma-inducing drug, as too much time had passed since they had stopped administering it. I had a sickening feeling something more was wrong.

'Look, we're concerned about his neurology,' explained Dr C. 'We're heart and lung specialists here, but I think it would be best if he was somewhere where there are experts in consciousness and comas. He should be at a hospital where neurologists are treating him, where the experts are on hand, not dialling in once a day to speak to us. I have a place in mind, Queen Square, but it's full and we can't get him in. We'll keep trying.'

By now Derek was testing negative for Covid. The virus had passed through his system, but that was of little comfort as the damage it had wreaked was horrific. It helped in one way, though: a place was available in a hospital in north

London that worked closely with the National Hospital for Neurology and Neurosurgery in Queen Square, sharing experts and expertise, but it would only take patients who were Covid-free. At last, some luck.

The team sedated him again for transfer. Another journey across London, unconscious and alone, on kidney dialysis and with machines monitoring all of his organs and a ventilator keeping him alive. Another worrying wait for him to arrive. I felt exhausted and anxious about having to get to know an entirely new set of specialists.

Hours after he left the heart and lung hospital, a doctor called, a new voice reassuring me that he had arrived safely but warning he was still very sick. He wanted to run a whole range of different tests and scans and would call when he knew more.

While this move to specialist treatment felt like a huge step forward, there remained the ever-present threat that Derek could die at any moment. Every day was frightening. Every day felt like a battle. Every day felt like wading further into the unknown. Each question answered even slightly evasively was rocket fuel to my anxieties. And, as it turned out, not without good reason.

On a Friday night, at 10.30 p.m., a doctor called, whom I had never spoken to before. He introduced himself, then said, 'Right. I have a question for you. What is your greatest fear?'

'Well, I don't know what you mean,' I replied. I didn't understand, why was he talking in riddles? What I really wanted to say was, 'Please don't play games.'

'What is your greatest fear?' he repeated.

'Well, that he dies. I mean, while there's life there's hope so my greatest fear must be that he dies.'

'Right. Well, I'm going to give you a second greatest fear. That he never changes from this.'

What did he mean? My mind raced.

'I mean that he stays like this, paralysed, including his face, unable to talk, unable to show any response at all, simply opening his eyes and closing them. He is still incredibly, incredibly sick.'

My body became cold and clammy with panic. What was he saying?

'Look, Covid has ripped through his body from the top of his head to the tips of his toes. He may still die, but even if he lives we have no idea if he can recover from this, from where he is now.'

So all of this time I had been praying for Derek to live, willing him to come home to us. Now I had this new, even more terrifying, fear that even if he lived he might still be lost.

Chapter 7

A Reckoning

A few days later I was waiting outside Derek's new hospital for a meeting with the team of specialists who would be looking after him. I hadn't left the house for weeks so hadn't seen anyone face to face, apart from my children. The thought of the outside world would have been completely overwhelming even without the prospect of a meeting that was making me nauseous with anxiety.

I still hadn't seen Derek since that initial brief visit to the hospital before he was rendered unconscious, and I hadn't seen his friend Ben Wegg-Prosser for much longer. I had asked Ben to come with me to this meeting, to provide not just moral support but a second pair of ears as I suspected that the information we would be discussing might be complicated, upsetting and potentially overwhelming. I wasn't sure I would be able to remember everything that was said if I was the only one there. Ben and I had been talking so intensely all of this time, but without being able to meet. Now, as he approached, I felt as if I was seeing a fantasy figure rather than someone real – as if Santa were walking towards me on a sunny early-summer day.

We both burst into tears – the sight of each other, the intensity of the emotion: just being outside in the world now felt so alien to us. I realized that Ben wasn't doing any socializing either, that we were all going through this weird national loneliness together. It was so wonderful to see him in the flesh but it made the reason we were meeting more piercingly real: it had given the jeopardy flesh. The instinct to give him a big hug, to thank him for everything, was so strong, but of course I couldn't, so we were reduced to nodding and smiling, wiping our tears from two metres apart before we headed into the hospital.

The room we sat in was the sort of temporary meeting space that no one finds welcoming. There was something so impersonal, so temporary about the desk and chairs, the anonymous art on the walls. It was exactly the kind of room where I imagined bad news was delivered. I wondered how many others had sat there waiting to know their fate. I didn't want to be there. And when I look back on this meeting now, it's almost as if I *wasn't* there. I felt as if I was watching CCTV or hearing what was said reported back from afar. I had thought I was going to find out either good news or bad news – but the truth was that I would hear something in between.

There were four of us: Ben, me, Dr W, a neurologist, and

the doctor who had called me on Friday night to deliver the news that Derek might never progress from a coma-like state. Once we were all sitting down and had made the relevant introductions, Dr W called up a variety of scans on to the screen in the room, all of brains. First, we saw one of a normal, healthy brain. Then we saw one of Derek's. It was very obviously different.

It was hard to know what I was seeing, rather like the first time a newly pregnant friend shows you a baby scan – you know you're looking at a baby but have no idea where anything is or what on earth it could mean, so you say, 'Wow! Great! Thrilled for you!'

'What am I looking at?' I asked.

'Derek's brain,' he replied.

I resisted the urge to say, 'Clearly,' because, after all, the poor man didn't know me from Adam. How could he know that I felt as though the last few months I had been taking an Open University course in anatomy and Covid, and had been across more scans, charts and medical information than I ever thought possible? Of course I knew it was a brain: I just didn't know which bits were worrying and what it meant.

I now know that Dr W is considered a genius, the closest thing to the patron saint of brains you're ever likely to meet, and I'm very lucky he is involved in Derek's care. Back then we were finding our feet, working each other out. I asked him to talk me through what was fluid, what was brain cell, where the nerves connected to the body, and what the blobs on Derek's scan, which were not on the 'normal' one, actually meant. They were like fluffy white clouds floating in the top part of his head.

He then showed me CT scans that had been taken at the heart and lung hospital and overlaid them on one of Derek's MRI scans. CT scans show much less detail than MRIs and, of course, Derek hadn't been able to have an MRI while he was on ECMO.

'So, this is the area that concerned the doctors where he was before, and they were worried that it might indicate strokes or brain bleeds, but weren't sure. And the areas they were worried about exactly match the fluffy clouds on the MRI.'

'So what does that mean?' I asked. 'Has he had strokes and bleeds?'

'Well, he has had a small bleed but that isn't his problem. The fluffy clouds show us that at some point Derek has had Covid inflammation in the white matter of his brain.'

By now I knew from my research that inflammation could be treated. There were procedures such as plasma exchange and drugs such as steroids that would bring inflammation down in all areas of the body and help tissues heal. But this, they told me, was a unique historical event, a one-off splurge of inflammation, and the fact that it showed up in some form on the earlier CT scans from back in April meant it had happened right at the start when Derek was first on ECMO. Then all the focus had been on his lungs, and keeping him breathing.

'OK, so what does this mean?' I asked. My usual pragmatic self was swinging back into action. 'This sounds very bad. But let's move to the solution. What are we going to do about it?'

'Well, inflammation in the brain is very rare and, of course, Covid is very new, so I haven't seen inflammation in the brain from Covid before. But I have heard from colleagues across Europe that some are being reported – but too few and too recently, really only a matter of days ago, so we can't yet predict the recovery. What we do know is that right now Derek is not waking up from the coma so all we can deduce is that it's entirely possible that the effect of this inflammation could be one of the reasons why. He might stay like this for ever. But there is no data, no precedent to make a prediction. So we just don't know.'

That phrase again: 'don't know'. The room started to spin. Of course I knew that Covid caused inflammation – it was what had wreaked havoc throughout the rest of his body, but this was the first time it had been mentioned that it had gone into his brain.

'The good news is,' Dr W continued, 'that we know he is not "brain dead".'

They had already done electrical tests to show that there was still activity. And they knew that these signs of inflammation, whatever it was, had not gone into the spinal cord or the brain stem, which was also good news: if that had happened it was more likely that the connection from brain to body, to movement and action, would be permanently affected.

So why the negativity? Why the fear he might never wake up?

Dr W explained that even though his eyes would open and he would occasionally be tracking, following things around the room, it was not consistent. Sometimes he would look at where the sound was coming from, at others he would ignore it and stare into space, so they couldn't conclude he was 'intentionally' looking.

There was some movement in his right thumb, but it was unclear whether it was voluntary or involuntary. If they held his hand and asked him to squeeze, sometimes after a pause he would, but at others he wouldn't. Was it communication or was it the involuntary grab reflex, which we all have from birth?

I had no context for any of this, no understanding of how to place this information in the future of Derek's or my life. The doctors explained that even though MRI scans are amazing, they can still only show a fraction of the cells of which a brain is made up. They had to hope that the billions we couldn't see were unaffected and he wasn't *more* affected than was visible. They thought that the grey matter was intact. It was the white matter, the wiring, where the problem was, and specifically in the myelin, the body's version of that plastic coating that covers electrical wires. I knew from talking to a neurologist before, when the spectre of strokes and bleeds was first raised, that in layman's terms grey matter is where thought is formed – 'I want a cup of tea.' The white matter is the mechanism by which the brain sends a thousand signals at once to move the hand to switch the kettle on and reach for the teabags. So if Derek's myelin had been affected by inflammation, it could mean the signals were getting mixed up, misfiring.

A glimmer of hope? Did that mean Derek could still think? Still know us? Have memories? Even if he couldn't show them? Then the next second: Oh God, does that mean if, as they fear, he doesn't change from this he'll be 'locked in', trapped inside his body for ever? It's the stuff of nightmares. A kind of torture.

My brain was racing, wanting to take it in, but not sure what I was actually meant to be taking in. I was trying so hard to listen, my face calm, but I was like the classic swan that looks peaceful on the surface while paddling furiously below the water. I was trying to assess, without them realizing, what they were really telling me. *Are they telling me this is it? Or is this a case of them laying out the worst possible scenario?*

Again, I asked, 'So what does this mean?'

'It's a case of "wait and see",' they explained.

'But there must be something we can *do*. Not just more waiting, surely.'

A pause. The doctors looked at each other with a glance I didn't understand.

'Well, the usual treatment for inflammation in the white matter of the brain is steroids and plasma exchange. But it works best when used within the first seventy-two hours of the attack.'

Two of the treatments I had been begging for right from the beginning. I had uncovered that other countries had been using steroids and plasma exchange for Covid infection with positive results – not for the brain, of course, as no one was focused on that, but for the lungs.

Dr W continued, 'Usually we can get them into a patient quickly in those first crucial hours but no one could see those symptoms because Derek was already in an induced coma.'

'What about trying steroids *now*? What about trying plasma exchange *now*? Because, OK, it might be too late to help in the way it would have done months ago but can it do any *harm*? Isn't it worth a try?'

'Well, we will think about it. I'll talk to Dr L, who is the specialist in this area of neurology, and we'll review it.' The answer was as cautious as ever. 'It's not medically sound to give anyone any procedure or drugs if we don't have proof it will clinically help.'

I wanted to scream. In fact, I could hear myself screaming in my head.

Jesus Christ, it's not going to hurt, is it? Why be so cautious at this point? Everyone has been so cautious all the way along. And now we're in this mess …

I said, 'Do you think if we'd had steroids when I was begging for steroids, it might have prevented this?'

'Yes,' he said. 'Yes. But it might also have killed him. We will never know.'

I felt as though I was on a seesaw, unable to get angry or sad or frustrated or distressed because in each case there was an alternative reality in which he could simply have died. Weeks ago. Months. Every single person involved was now saying it was a miracle Derek had got this far, had lived this long. All the way through this process I'd been told that it was all about the lungs, that if we could get the lungs working, the kidneys, the liver and the heart would have a chance to recover. Now, suddenly, it seemed it was all about the brain.

'So is this his biggest problem for recovery now?' I asked.

There was a very, very long pause before he gave me his answer.

'Well, biologically, everything below the neck is really only there to support the brain. The reason we have legs is so we can hunt and get food to nourish our brain. Everything we do is really all about the brain ...'

He was being so philosophical. I didn't want to discuss the nature of the human: I wanted to be told statistics, drug names, treatment pathways – *cures*.

'The brain is always the slowest to recover,' he said, 'and, remember, he is still very, very sick. In a critical condition. His lungs, his kidneys, his heart, his liver, his pancreas are all needing massive support so there is an argument that all this will have to start recovering first before we can know more about the impact on the brain.'

'So, do you think a recovery is possible?' I pressed, desperate to get some sort of a straight answer out of him.

'We can't rule out some kind of recovery. But we can't rule out him never recovering.'

Somewhere among the double negatives in that sentence I was trying to extract a flicker of hope.

'What do you mean?' I asked, for what felt like the hundredth time.

'I think a good recovery would be exceptional – but I don't think, at this stage, we have the evidence to rule out a reasonable recovery.'

I needed some kind of scale: what was reasonable? Derek back home being Derek but maybe with a bit of a limp? In a wheelchair, with some short-term memory loss? With an inhaler or drugs for life?

'So, if the worst is that he doesn't change from now, and the best is that you can't rule out a "reasonable" recovery, what does a reasonable recovery look like? What is the best we can hope for? What is in your mind when you use that term?'

His reply was a phrase that still haunts me. 'Being able to hold a hairbrush.'

I felt as though I'd been shot.

That phrase seemed to summon images of damaged people sitting in institutions, with just one hand on a hairbrush, slowly brushing. It was the sort of picture you've seen in old-fashioned movies. That's what came to mind: black-and-white movies in which a character ends up 'in an institution'. Someone sitting in a chair, staring blankly out of the window.

It just went through me. It seemed a world away from anything I had ever associated with Derek. I had this pitiful scene in my head, but also the Derek I knew swirling alongside it. Derek – brilliantly clever, mentally terrifying in his incisive assessing of any situation, full of spirit and humour, and infuriating, constantly challenging. Never passive, never compliant. My sounding board, the yin to my yang, the inspirational father to my children, my love, my life.

Not only all that, but for so long the mind had literally been his job. The very thing he was brilliant at was assessing and *getting* people. Right from his early days of being in politics. After all, that's what politics is about. It's about people. It's about relationships. About minds. It's about motivation, energy, how to find what makes people tick and inspire them to do things. He had taught me so much about how the mind works and now … this?

I felt out of my body, floating somewhere above. The room became blisteringly bright and white. Was I going to faint? And the noise, the overwhelming noise: nothing specific, just an unbearable white sound that makes you desperate to cover your ears. I almost did but somehow I knew the room was actually silent, deadly silent in fact: it was all in my head.

I had the same experience in childbirth – in those final moments when you have to push with all your might, I felt I was bellowing, the midwife was screaming, the white noise was blaring, but when we watched the video Derek had made, I was so quiet. In fact, apart from the soft encouragement of the midwife to push, there was no noise at all. It was as if everything in my head was so loud, so vivid, that the room was just kind of blank, really still, really quiet, absorbing the roaring of my mind.

I don't know how long this moment went on for. I suppose it must have been seconds, but I felt as if I was travelling for days. As if I was walking across that rope bridge in the jungle from the life I had known to the life that was now facing me. Except when I faced the real rope bridge I had been calm. It's a TV show, I had told myself. Of course it's fine. You'll be fine.

Now, however, I had no such reassurances. I just had to take a breath and say to myself, OK, onwards. I just remember thinking, I need to know more. I need more detail.

I heard myself say as much.

Out of the corner of my eye, I became aware that Ben was also staring at Dr W, clearly in shock too, trying to grapple with this incredibly intense conversation.

'So if a good recovery is exceptional, does he have a chance of being the exception?' He was clearly trying to probe for something positive, something hopeful to take out of this. It felt as if every time I tried to find a way to move forward to search out a pathway, a treatment, Dr W was blocking it. Later, once we had got to know each other better, he explained that was what the meeting was about – and that it was incredibly painful for doctors too. The point was brutally to lay out the facts at Ground Zero. To try to get the family to see the reality of where Derek was right now. To explain only what the neurologist could be confident was true and what he could deliver. He couldn't talk about a glimmer of hope he wasn't confident about in case the family – me – might take that glimmer and spiral off into false hope. By stating only the facts as they were right then, he was taking me to my lowest ebb, so that he could begin to work with Derek from there. I understood it was the right way to do it but for me it was like receiving knock-out blow after knock-out blow.

'Obviously if he were the exception I would be delighted,' Dr W said, almost as if he sensed that the relentless negativity, the relentless stripping away of hope was turning him into the bad guy – it was as if he was saying, 'Be reassured,

I don't *want* this to be the case, I just have to get you to where I am.' I felt as if I had seen the first flicker of humanity, of human emotion. Everything had been so scientific, but also strangely imprecise, scientific scans showing something the effect of which wasn't truly known. Blobs on a screen that could mean so much, yet confirmed so little. I felt I was trying to divine my future from tea leaves when I looked at them.

And just at this point, the other doctor piped up, seeming to take up the slack. 'There is always hope,' he explained. 'We don't know everything about the human body and the brain particularly is still a huge mystery, even to experts like Dr W.'

My head spun around to pay more attention to this guy. It was as if he'd just walked into the room with an ice cream. A steaming cup of tea and an ice cream, just for me.

'There is always hope,' he repeated. 'The first thing you're taught at medical school is never say never, and never say always. So you never say, "This person is never going to recover." And you never say, "From this condition or situation someone always recovers." Because the human body can always surprise you. So that is hope, and hope is really important.'

It felt as if the air in the room was changing as he looked at me, really hard. It was as if he was willing me to pick up on this.

Buoyed, I swung back to Dr W. 'Have you had anyone with scans showing this kind of impact before, not just with Covid because I know that's new, but with any kind of inflammation? Anyone who's made a good recovery? Have you ever seen effects on a brain like this before?'

He paused for a long time. 'No,' he replied. 'But – and it's a big but – I have never seen anything like this before so can't personally chart the recovery. It's very, very unusual and generally only seen in children, who can often make a good recovery. To see it in an adult is extremely rare and from Covid it has not really been seen at all because the virus itself is so new. So we just don't know. We don't have anything to measure it against.' Then he looked down and, almost under his breath, said sadly, 'He is very, very unlucky.'

Then Ben, who had been sitting quietly, looking shell-shocked for the whole meeting, spoke up again. 'So … there *is* hope?' he said, heartbreakingly softly, almost like a little boy. 'There is hope that Derek could be the exception because Derek *has* always been an exception …'

'Well, that's right for sure,' I chimed in. 'He's been an exception all his life, sometimes exceptionally great. Sometimes exceptionally ridiculous.' I smiled at Ben, comforted by someone in the room who knew Derek and understood the affection in what I meant by 'ridiculous'. 'He's never followed the *usual* path in anything.'

'Well, to give you some context on just how often we can get surprised,' Dr W continued, 'I've been dealing recently with a man who for seven months hadn't moved at all, not even a flicker or twitch, nothing. There'd been no response whatsoever, not even opening his eyes as Derek is. And just a couple of weeks ago he started to move and to respond. For seven months, there'd been no response. Seven!'

'Is it the same problem as Derek?' Ben asked.

'No, he's a soldier and had been shot in the head.'

Later Ben told me he had been absolutely floored by this response. He just couldn't believe that Derek, who had had a virus that we'd been told attacks the lungs, was being compared to somebody who had taken a gunshot to the head.

So I asked what we all wanted to: 'Is this man now going to be OK?'

Dr W looked at me for what seemed like a lifetime. It definitely was a long time, as all of these scientists leave about forty seconds before each response, while they think carefully about what *precisely* the right answer might be. Then out came two words.

'Not really.'

I was desperate, thirsty for just something, anything to grab hold of here. Why were they all being so closed?

'Dr W, you've got to expand more. Use more words! Use more words! I can't stand this!' It was the closest I had come to exploding in emotion, because it was just too painful. It felt like trying to draw blood out of a stone.

'What I mean is,' he continued, 'it's highly unlikely that man will return to the way he was before. But Derek's situation is different because we don't yet know how Covid inflammation will affect him. I only use it as an example of how someone in the hospital where he was being treated had been completely written off, yet started to recover with no explanation. And no change in treatment. Just time. Time and waiting are your friends here.'

I had already waited so long.

'How long before you know more? Not how long will it take for him to recover, because you don't know if he can even recover, but how long before you might know more?'

It was a confusing question, but I knew what I meant and he seemed to as well. After another long pause, he looked straight at me, then away.

'Well, Kate' – the first time he had used my name – 'I think it's fair to say if he is still like this after two years we will know there is very little chance of him making any meaningful recovery.'

TWO YEARS!

I screamed inside my head. Up until now I had been living by the minute, hours on the phone monitoring infection levels and statistics, trying to get a handle on where Derek was, wondering every time I went to sleep if he would still be alive in the morning. How could I go on like this for another two years? Worse still, how could Derek be trapped like this for *two years*? The timescale winded me and I'm sure I must have slumped a bit in the chair.

The other doctor seemed to sense this and said carefully, 'What you have to get your head around, Kate, is that you're now moving to a different phase. Dr W is a neurologist. I am an intensive-care specialist with thirty years' experience and I see this all the time. For a while families of patients who are very sick live on a knife edge, fearing they might die. This is what we doctors call the acute phase for the patient. Then they slightly improve and the families breathe a huge sigh of relief, but actually the long, slow recovery is sometimes just as hard to bear. We call this the chronic phase. The hard thing for you is that you're going to have to live through both phases at the same time. Derek is still very sick, at serious risk of dying. But even if he can live, and begin to recover from the huge damage Covid has wreaked throughout his body, it's not going to be quick. Progress is now going to be measured not in minutes, hours or days but in weeks, months and years. And you are going to have to bear that journey never knowing if he might ever be the person he was before, knowing he might never truly come back to you. You just have to give us time and be strong.'

I sensed they were trying to wrap things up. But I couldn't take in what they were saying. I wanted space to take it in. I didn't want to wrap up on this level of bleakness.

'You mentioned a specialist, Dr L, I think,' I added. 'Can you connect me with him please?' I wanted to have someone else to ask things of, someone who was an expert to process it with. Dr W looked a little offended. 'Not because I don't trust everything you're saying, by the way. This is not a second-opinion situation. It's just such a lot to take in and it would be good to have someone else to talk to and to learn more.'

'Well, I'm not sure if he'll speak to you – he doesn't generally. He feeds information through the neurologist in charge, me. But I will talk to him and ask him. I will also talk to him about the steroids and plasma exchange and will call you next week with what we've decided.'

Even waiting until the next week seemed too long, a week just to know the next step. But by now they were on their feet and our time was clearly up. I mumbled something about being sorry to keep them because I knew how much pressure they were under, with so many people sick, thanked them for their time and said a dazed goodbye.

We were ushered into a little side room while they went to fetch a nurse from the area of the hospital where Derek was. I had been asked to bring some things in for his room, some pictures and trinkets that he might be able to see, might make him feel at home, and they could study any reaction.

It was only that morning, but it seemed a lifetime ago that I had been putting together a big bag of photographs of the children and us as a family, a couple of ornaments from Derek's study, and a large brightly coloured wall-hanging from his Thinking Room. I figured that as we didn't know how much he could see, the bigger and more distinctive the better. It had seemed a lovely thing to do, a way of getting closer to him, even though I couldn't see him. Now, in just an intensive hour and a half, everything had changed, and he felt further away than ever. I almost couldn't bear to give them these personal things. Suddenly it felt like acknowledgement that he was in for longer than I could imagine, an acceptance of separation.

It was torture sitting there, knowing that we were only a couple of floors away from where he was, but not allowed to go and see him, to hug him, to tell him he was going to be all right, even though I didn't know whether he would or ever could be. Now, when I was the nearest I had been to him since he first got sick, I felt further away than ever before.

When the nurse arrived, I could tell she was doing her best to bridge the gap between me on the ground floor and

Derek a few flights up. She looked at the bits I had brought, saying to me that they were brilliant and would really help.

'Oh, this is all great,' she told me. 'I'll send you a photo of how we've arranged them in the room.'

But all I could do was to smile bleakly and thank her. I didn't want a photograph of Derek. I wanted Derek.

We had to leave, our restricted time was up, but neither of us wanted to go. We loitered limply outside, two metres apart, struggling to find a way of not letting the bleak 'wait and see' simply be *it*.

'How do you feel about how that went?' I asked Ben.

'Pretty bad,' he replied.

'Yeah, me too.'

Then a silence, neither of us really knowing what to say to help the other, but not really wanting to go.

'Look, we'll just have to make sure he is the exception,' he said. 'We'll keep researching. We'll find something to make him the exception. We won't give up. None of us.'

'OK,' I said. 'I'll focus on getting hold of Dr L.'

'And I'll focus on Lucian Grainge,' he replied.

Sir Lucian was a friend of Sir Elton John and the global Chairman of Universal Music. Coincidentally Ben and another friend of mine knew him too. He had had coronavirus back in early March, had been dangerously sick and even been put into a coma like Derek. But he was now well on the road to recovery. It had been a long haul: as he came round out of the induced coma he was profoundly confused due to the impact of the medication and after effects of Covid. His recovery was tough and had taken its toll but he was getting there. Maybe he could shed some light on what we had just heard.

'And I'm going to look into contacts in Israel as well,' he added.

It sounded left field but actually made sense. Israel, tragically, was now known for pioneering work on brain recovery, because of the decades of conflict in the region and the inevitable head injuries.

We both started to feel strength returning, hope surging.

There was a plan. I wasn't prepared to accept that this was it, until somebody could confidently tell me otherwise. Not just because it was so horrific to consider but because accepting it meant giving up on Derek, acquiescing to things being out of our hands. It would have felt like leaving him in no man's land. At the very least, we had to try to carry him back to the trench to give him our best. As Ben and I said our goodbyes to each other that day, we reassured each other: 'We've got to do this. We've got to hope. We've at least got to try.'

Of course we weren't leaving him in no man's land: he was with extraordinary health-care professionals who were doing everything they could. If anyone was going to get him out of no man's land it would be them. But somehow having a plan of what *we* could do helped to ease the sense of helplessness, the agony of 'wait and see'. But, really, the enormity of what we had just been through hadn't fully sunk in: we were still in shock and the true reality of the fight that lay ahead was still to come.

Chapter 8

Shock

I felt numb in the taxi heading home. Shock had hit me so many times, following so many frightening phone calls since Derek had first become ill, that I could recognize it and knew how it affected me, but this was different. It was like shock had a new face. This time, the familiarity of having been through it before didn't help me. This shock was a stranger.

The new disaster I had been presented with – Derek lost for ever, locked in a perpetual state of semi-consciousness – was too big to process. Before, it had been live or die, on or off. Binary. So I had been swinging between two extremes of emotion: joy at the chance of him living, fear of the tsunami of grief at him dying. Back and forward, back and forward, every second of every minute of every hour of the day. And I had learnt how to manage that terror, to control that adrenalin, at least enough to function. Now, it wasn't just on or off, back or forward. I was swinging three ways, spinning out of control.

And the vastness of the time – *two years* – was like a black hole. There was nothing to get any purchase on, no date on a calendar to aim for. No reassuring sentence to myself: 'Just get through today, Kate, and pray he doesn't die.' *Two years* before I would know if he was still 'in there', before I would know if he really could live. Two years before I would know whether there was any kind of future. How could I plan? How could I hope? And how could I get a handle on this?

I tried to wrestle my thoughts into order. 'Right. Well, Ben Wegg-Prosser and I have a plan,' I told myself. That settled me a bit, even though I knew I was in no fit state to start enacting it right now. 'Tomorrow,' I told myself.

Usually I would call Derek's family directly after a big meeting, phone call or development to keep them in the loop. Right from the beginning I had made the decision that I would always be honest with them. I felt that I didn't have the right to withhold anything, even with the best of intentions to try to protect them from further hurt and distress. I knew if it was my child or brother I would want to know everything, and I believed that they had to as well. But there was still a balance to be maintained between keeping them informed and dumping my worries on them when I was having a bad day. That just felt like scaremongering, especially as the doctors were faced with so many 'don't knows' themselves. I also tried always to bear in mind that they were hundreds of miles away. They hadn't seen Derek since he'd got sick, not even the snatched FaceTime that I had had. Derek's mum didn't have a tablet or an iPhone so they felt helpless, drowning in the same anxieties and fears as me but so far away. Before I could decide what to do, Derek's mum called me. She knew I'd had a meeting at the hospital, and had been on pins waiting to hear.

'What did they say? How are his lungs? What are his blood-oxygen levels?'

Like me she had started to write down the details, the crumbs of facts given out by whichever nurse or doctor I got through to each day. I had passed on the numbers, seemingly random at first, and now she, too, was using them to measure any flicker of progress. I suddenly realized that in that meeting, for the first time in a long time, I hadn't asked about any of that. The new fear had swept those details entirely away. Understandably, Derek's mum was still locked in the mantra we had been given by his previous doctors: *It's all about the lungs. It's all about the lungs.*

'Well, they didn't really mention the lungs,' I said gently. 'One of the intensive-care doctors *was* at the meeting, but it was really being led by a neurologist because now their greater worry is why he isn't coming out of the coma, and how Covid might have affected Derek's brain and nervous system.'

'What – strokes and bleeds?'

'No,' I said. 'It seems they aren't the problem, although I know previous scans had suggested they might be there. It seems that just as Derek's immune response to the Covid virus has caused inflammation in his body, which has affected and damaged his lungs, heart, liver and kidneys, it might also have affected the wiring in his brain. It could be why he can't wake up from the coma.'

A long silence.

'So his immune response to the Covid, his body's fight against the disease, has done the damage?'

I explained what I had been told: that when the body reacts to a virus like Covid, it tries to attack the disease: the immune response. But in some cases the immune system overreacts, and when it can't contain the virus, infection starts to attack everything, including healthy cells, which causes more inflammation that leads to more damage. And this was what had happened in Derek's case.

'So,' she asked, 'by fighting off the disease so hard, by his immune response to Covid, he could be left like this for ever?'

In a way, she was right.

'Yes, but remember if his body hadn't fought so hard, as you put it, he might be dead, like so many others. He is still here. He is still alive.'

'Where there's life there's hope,' I heard her murmur under her breath. Then another long silence. I knew she was winded. I imagined her, frail, thin, shredded to almost nothing by months of terror.

In the background Derek's dad was shouting – clearly I had been on speakerphone. 'He'll be all right, our Derek. He won't stay stuck in that coma – he'll find a way out. He's got a brain the size of a planet. He'll be fine.'

It was heartbreaking.

I knew they had an image of Derek as they'd last seen

him, at Christmas. Loud and full of life, cracking jokes and teasing them, driving our nieces and nephews mad with ludicrous mimes in charades. How could they visualize him as he was now? Silent, expressionless, all that life trapped inside a body that was devastated.

'I talk to him every morning you know,' Derek's dad, Ken, continued, closer to the phone now.

'You talk to him?' I asked, wondering if he'd managed to get through on the phone to talk to him in his unconscious state, the nurses holding the phone to his ear as they had been doing for me.

'No, no, not on the phone. Just father to son. We have a connection. I just go out with a brew into our backyard and I talk to him, man to man like. I tell him he's got everything to fight for. A wife that loves him, two kids he'd do anything for. He'll pull through. He'll be back, Kate. I just know it – I can *feel* it.'

The tears were flowing down my cheeks now, but I didn't make a sound. The love he felt was real enough, the connection, too, I'm sure, but who was he connected to? Did that person even exist any more? Was he deluding himself to hang on to a false reality, to hang on to hope? Was I, too?

'How long before the doctors know?' Derek's mum, Chrina, interrupted, yanking me out of my thoughts.

'Well, they don't know how long before they'll know ...' I almost laughed at how insanely unhelpful that sounded. I knew that, like me, she was scrabbling for something to hang on to. 'But it will be a long time. He has so much to recover from. He's still so weak and is running another temperature.'

181

Throughout this time he had been getting lots of other infections, bacterial ones that fortunately, unlike Covid, could be treated with antibiotics. At one point he even had bacterial pneumonia, enough on its own to land someone in hospital, and he had it *on top* of coronavirus.

'Oh, of course they don't know. They don't know Derek and they don't know this virus.' Derek's dad had joined in again. 'They thought he was going to die weeks, months ago and he didn't. He'll show them, Kate, you mark my words. He'll show them – he won't stay like this for long. He won't stay in that coma, believe me, Kate.'

He was getting louder, more determined, more convinced. It was the rallying cry of a man who'd seen and heard so-called 'experts', and what he would call 'more educated men', be wrong before. A war cry, from a man who had grown up on the canals where his dad had worked as a 'legger', back when horses drew the boats carrying coal from the mines. When the long boats went through the bridges, the towpath ran out, and the horse – a precious commodity as it was the power source – would be walked over the bridge.

William Draper, Derek's granddad – whom Bill is named after – would lie down on a plank hanging over the side of the boat and, with his feet against the inner side of the bridge, use his legs to 'walk' the boat through. It was one of Derek's biggest working-class prides that his granddad had worked so hard to give his family of twelve kids a chance in life, even if he always boasted about it in his usual taking-the-mick way. When he was in a fancy London restaurant with his so-called 'posh friends', he would say, 'My granddad was lower in the socio-economic status of his community than a horse. Basically he was a horse's back-up! An assistant to a horse!' Then he would raise a glass of expensive champagne and say, with a wink, 'In two generations I've not done badly, have I?'

Derek's dad, Ken, loved learning, but like so many of his generation, with money so tight at home, he had left school at fourteen to go 'down the pit', the main source of work in the area. His job then was to carry the thick, heavy blocks of wood down to the experienced miners who used them to shore up the tunnels. It must have been dark, claustrophobic, frightening work for a young lad who loved climbing hills and running wild with his brothers and sisters in the nearby sprawling countryside. But when I've asked him about it, he only ever says, 'It was OK because the men down there made it OK. They looked out for each other, you know. And they looked after me. Yes, they would constantly be joking, the banter kept us all going, but when the chips were down they would look out for each other. They were there for each other.'

He told us all about one time when a tunnel collapsed and some of the men were buried under piles of rock and coal. They could hear their screams but couldn't get to them. The men Ken was with kept shouting, 'Don't worry, we'll get you out, you'll be all right.' But he said he saw the fear on their faces as they scrabbled with their tools, their bare hands – anything – desperate to free them.

'I'll never forget that day, watching, trying to help as much as I could, as they fought so hard, their hands cut to ribbons from the rocks, bleeding but not even noticing. They managed it, though,' Ken said. 'We got all three of them out and dragged them, black, bruised, bleeding and choking, to the surface. And I tell you what, Kate. It wasn't the clever structural engineers who had calculated weight ratios that got them out, or the bosses with their degrees, it was grit, fight and never letting your friends down that got them out.'

All this came back to me as Ken carried on talking to me on the phone, shouting now: 'What do doctors know? It's not their fault but they're as clueless against Covid as the rest of us. Their experience counts for nothing.'

And suddenly he didn't seem delusional. Maybe we couldn't face up to reality – because what *was* the reality we were supposed to be facing up to? There were no hard facts and too many 'don't knows'. When science and experience are no longer solid, why not depend on the foundation of grit, striving, love and, yes, hope? After all, wasn't it the same grit that was keeping the doctors and nurses working long after their shifts had ended, battling an unknown and invisible enemy to keep Derek alive?

I looked out of the taxi window and realized we weren't moving. We had pulled up outside my home and the driver, who could perhaps see my tears over the top of my mask, or had maybe picked up on the sensitivity of the conversation, hadn't wanted to interrupt.

'Sorry, I didn't notice we'd arrived.'

'Don't worry, love, you take your time.'

As I scrambled to pay, I saw the curtains at the bedroom

window pull back. Darcey and Bill were peering out anxiously, knowing they weren't allowed to answer the door, but clearly wondering why I wasn't coming in.

Never mind what the future might hold, I knew what Derek would have been telling me in that moment. *Our love for each other is the only reality you need right now, Kate, so get some grit, go in and smother them with enough love for the both of us.*

The next day a useful distraction came in the shape of three enormous Amazon boxes. Like the rest of the country, we had been ordering everything online for months. We still hadn't been out to the shops, and home deliveries seemed impossible to arrange, so other than 'rescue packages' from friends and family, I had taken to ordering all the boring practicals like loo roll, bleach and socks (where do they disappear to?) with a click of a button. I had learnt to my cost that it's all too easy to think you're ordering three bottles of bleach, only to find you've ordered three crates, and we'd already had a few hilarious moments when enough washing powder to clean the entire British Navy's whites had turned up one day – all in one go! But even with my technical incompetence, the boxes that had just arrived seemed ridiculously huge.

'What have you done now?' Darcey said, as we struggled to drag them in across the doorstep.

The scoffing quickly turned to screams of delight when we discovered that they were three huge gymnastic blocks that Derek and I had tried to get hold of just before lockdown, and a large sponge floor mat. Derek loved setting up obstacle courses for the kids in the garden: things to leap over and run round as they competed against each other to go higher, faster, longer, while he timed them.

But as they had got older, just jumping through a hoop or sprinting backwards and forwards hadn't cut the mustard any more, so as we saw lockdown approaching and knew we would be spending a lot of time in the garden, we had ordered these. Obviously loads of other people had had the same idea, as they had been out of stock for weeks. What a perfect time for them to arrive. It was lovely to watch Darcey and Bill building towers, climbing up, leaping over and collapsing into fits of giggles.

Then the cardboard boxes came into play. We dragged out all the previous ones that hadn't made it into recycling and built a huge 'box fort'. Cue two hours of Nerf-gun battles …

'This is so cool,' Bill said. 'Will you film it for Dad? You can show him when he's better.'

It was as though Dad was here with us, part of our fun.

They were so happy and involved I even managed to nip inside and leave them for a bit to get some washing done and have a clear-up. It felt good to be doing something normal and domestic, I thought, as I put the clothes away. Although, as I looked out of the bedroom window and spotted the garden, I did pity our neighbours. On both sides the elderly couples are keen gardeners and weeks of shielding at home meant they had had time to make their gardens immaculate. They were neatness and perfection, while ours was now strewn with cascading cardboard boxes and bits of foam from the Nerf battle. To be honest, it looked like a giant recycling centre. I felt almost giddy with the relief of having a moment of silliness, laughing at the ridiculousness of what we had to do to get through, and how that must have appeared to others. I was still laughing when the phone rang.

'Hello?' I answered perkily, almost forgetting the dread that phone calls could now bring.

'Oh, you sound happy. It's Dr W here,' he said.

On hearing his voice I immediately sobered up.

'What news? Is he still alive?'

'Yes, yes, absolutely, and I have some news that I think you'll be pleased about. We've had a meeting and we're going to put him on a course of the steroids, and do the plasma exchange you were wanting us to do.'

'Well, only if it's right for him, Dr W,' I said, reeling slightly at '*you* were wanting'. 'You're the experts. I'm sorry, I know I can be a bit of a battering ram, but it's only because I've felt I had to be. I don't want you to feel under pressure to do things that I want if it's not right in your expert opinion.'

'No, don't worry, we totally understand the battering-ram thing. You've had so much frustration because Derek has always been just ahead of the curve, in the wrong way. As we doctors in all disciplines have been struggling to get on top of what this Covid actually is, Derek has always been just too late to benefit – so far.'

I liked the sound of 'so far'.

'But if it's any comfort to you at all, looking at the damage

Covid has done to Derek *will* help others. We're learning all the time, and it's looking at severe examples like this that effect change in practice. I was asked to ask you if you would consider allowing him to be recruited on to a new trial, called the recovery trial, so that we can learn from him.'

I said yes immediately, not just because I knew Derek would want it, liking the idea he was contributing to a greater sum of knowledge, but also because I felt anything was better than the 'wait and see' approach. 'Promise me one thing, though. He won't be some kind of control experiment, will he? You will actually give him treatment that you believe may help him to recover?'

He explained that the recovery trial was more of a monitoring than a testing situation. The doctors and specialists treating Derek would always put his recovery as the ultimate priority, do what they believed to be best. And it was an entirely separate team that would collect the results of his trial, which would be collated with others. Months later I now know that this trial has been really helpful to doctors and new patients right across the country, so I'm glad I said yes and hope to share that with Derek one day too.

But for now it was only Derek's recovery that filled my mind.

Dr W said he had had a meeting with a radiographer to look at Derek's scans in detail, and one with Dr L, whom he had mentioned in our first meeting. The radiographer said it wasn't clear that steroids and plasma exchange would be effective, but the other two had thought it worth a go.

'Steroids suppress the immune system, to stop it

over-responding and causing damage, which can be unhelpful, but in this case if there is still active inflammation it will
help to reduce it. Plasma exchange takes out the "bad stuff"
from the blood and puts clean plasma back in,' continued
Dr W. 'It will be at least two weeks before the course of
steroids and the process of plasma exchange is complete.
It usually works quickly but as we're in the world of the
unknown it could well take longer. So you're going to have
to be patient. And be prepared for it to be too late to have
any significant effect.'

I asked if they were any closer to knowing what the scans
showed and he said they thought they were – and then he
used a term that sounded like 'Aydem'.

'How do you spell that?' I asked, scrambling for a pen.

'It's an acronym. ADEM: acute disseminated encephalo-
myelitis. Acute means severe and disseminated means
widespread, scattered, not focused on one spot. Encephalo
relates to inflammation, and myelitis because it's in the
white matter of the brain, the connecting wiring that links
the grey matter to the body.

'But don't get hung up on that,' he went on. 'It's only an
umbrella term covering inflammation in that area. It doesn't
really give us any clues as to what exactly has happened and
how to cure it.'

We parted, with him saying that Dr L would call me soon
to explain more but, despite his warning not to "get hung
up" on it I, of course, immediately googled 'ADEM'.

The first entry to come up described it as 'A rare kind of
immune response causing inflammation, affecting the brain,

spinal cord and nerves, usually in children, often following a viral or bacterial infection. Symptoms include extreme fatigue, headache, and nausea.'

God, Derek had all of these, and he had never had the 'temperature and continuous cough', the main symptoms we were all told to look out for at the start of the Covid outbreak. Again, I cursed how much focus had been put on those. If we had known more back then, maybe I could have got him treatment sooner. But nobody had known back then, so I pushed away the unhelpful regret and focused on the more hopeful following sentence: 'Symptoms, though severe, are treatable. Most people make a full recovery and don't have another attack.' That sounded a lot more positive.

The next phone call with any news came later that day, from the lead intensive-care consultant in charge of Derek's care. I immediately asked him about ADEM, to which he said, 'Let me stop you there. Dr W and the other neurologists are in charge of Peedoc.'

'Peedoc?' I queried.

'Sorry, it's an acronym – PDOC.'

Yet more letters.

'Prolonged Disorder Of Consciousness. Basically, if someone doesn't come round from a coma quickly in the first few days, they have a consciousness disorder. If it goes on longer than usual, it's "prolonged". That is the category which Derek is now under. It's an umbrella term.'

God, Derek now had so many umbrella terms covering him, why did I feel they were doing nothing to shelter him from this storm?

'So the neurologists who are experts in that field will be in charge of drawing him out of the disorder of consciousness. That all comes under neurology,' he continued, 'while I and the other intensive-care doctors focus on everything else that's going on in the body, and how it might be impacting on his recovery, on him waking up. Because so little is known about what Covid does, we now have to rule out every other disease or infection so we can really understand the long-term damage to his body. He's still at risk of dying, he's still critical. Let's not forget that. So we need to look at how his heart has been affected – for example, he now has a hole in it. How his lungs are a long way away from breathing completely on their own, how he is still running infections throughout his body. His muscles are wasted to almost nothing. We have to establish whether that is simply because they haven't been moved for so long and are so weak, or whether something else is preventing him from activating them, and whether that is why he's paralysed.'

'Could the paralysis be permanent?' The thought of Derek trapped for ever, unable to move even his face muscles, was again filling my mind.

'We don't know,' came the response. 'But if you think about it, he also has to recover from the "cure" as well as the disease. ECMO itself is hugely traumatic to the body, especially all his blood vessels, and we're concerned that where the tubes were in his legs for so long, it's tough for the entry points to heal. Derek has been having bleeds from there, and we're worried about infections developing in those areas, which could then spread to the rest of his body.

We know he has clots in his lungs, and Heaven forfend that they should develop anywhere else because they could travel through the bloodstream and cause more damage. He has been on very high doses of a broad range of antibiotics for months, which have been necessary, but can also lay the system low, and are not helpful to the intestines and stomach. We are concerned that he is not absorbing the liquid food he is being fed through his nose and down into his stomach. He is not opening his bowels and is still losing weight, so that might indicate a failure to absorb. It certainly shows that something is not functioning properly and, please God, we need to find out what. We also need to look at his liver and pancreas. They are not working well, and he wasn't Type 1 diabetic before this, so why is he suddenly not able to produce enough insulin to control his blood sugars now? His kidneys are on full dialysis, and we know that can affect neurology, so it might be contributing to him staying in this semi-conscious state. It might simply be that because the kidneys use so much oxygen to function, and his lungs have been struggling to get oxygen in, that they have just shut down – a kind of body self-preservation so that the precious oxygen can go to where it's most needed. It could be that as the rest of his body starts to recover, please God, the kidneys will too. We do see that in intensive care. It's not unusual. Or it could be that something else is affecting his kidneys. It's my job to go through everything, check every single thing, to see if something *else* is hindering his recovery, and to hope that, please God, it's something we can treat. And even if nothing but Covid damage is affecting him, then at least we can confidently rule out all other avenues of medical help.'

His passion was touching. The use of hope and so many 'please God's felt human, as if he, too, was willing Derek back. It was also shocking, the scale of what Derek and the team were up against and the size of the challenge ahead.

I did what friends will know I often do when things are overwhelmingly bleak: I reached for an inappropriate joke, silliness, anything to break the tension.

'Crikey, you sound like you're some kind of medical Poirot, detecting your way round Derek's body trying to use your "little grey cells" to find the culprit threatening his life!'

It instantly comforted me. Poirot is my go-to comfort telly. There's something about that era, the beauty of the art-deco style, the furniture Derek and I had filled our home with. I have always found Poirot's cleverness soothing, and his eccentricity hilarious. Plus, he always managed to wrap up the most dastardly of deeds and end the show neatly, with everyone happy and laughing. That's the kind of drama I felt I could do with right now, rather than the unending unsolvable bleakness of the one I was facing in reality.

My comment might have gone wrong – he might have seen me as flippant and nothing else. But, thankfully, he laughed, perhaps relieved, too, to have a break in the tension, the relentlessly miserable stream of information.

'Well, yes,' he said, 'although I don't think the moustache would suit me! But if I'm a Poirot, you have to help too. I need you to be a Miss Marple. I need you to tell me every ailment Derek has had, anything you know about where he might have travelled to over the years. What sicknesses he had in his childhood, what bugs he might have picked up abroad. The more you can find out the better.'

It felt good to be able to contribute, to be part of the team, rather than simply asking questions to which they had no answers. Now maybe *I* could find out some answers. So I busied myself trying to get to the bottom of Derek's story, talking to his mum and dad, his sisters, his friends and anyone he had travelled with for work, hoping to find a clue that would help the doctors.

It made me realize that, while the medics were working so hard, there was still a huge amount for Derek's family, friends and me to do. I felt it was going to be a process of hauling him back – all of us would have to play our part. Derek needed to know that we were there, waiting, that we wanted him and loved him, and that we were all on his team. So the following week Ben and I got down to business. I even managed to get hold of Dr L, the brain-inflammation specialist neurologist.

'There are four or five people I've seen so far, from the sharing we're doing nationally and across Europe, who seem to be showing the effects on their scans that Derek is displaying. But I fear we will see more. There are similarities to the ADEM we have seen over the years but there are also differences. One man actually looks slightly worse than Derek, but in behavioural terms he's doing much better. He is already much more conscious, much more awake, much more responsive. And that is the problem with working from scans – there is too much about the brain that you just can't see. So Derek could be more affected in a way that we can't see. But that opens up equal opportunity for recovery that we might not predict. I think a good recovery, again, *would* be exceptional. But also … why not? The whole point of exceptions is someone has got to be one – so why not Derek?'

This was an attitude I could work with. He kept on talking about Covid ADEM and I realized immediately that the words just needed to run together. 'CoviDEM is now what you specialize in, then?'

'Yes! And that's a good word for it.'

'Well, you can have it – I'm all give! At last I've contributed something, Dr L, instead of just asking awkward questions!'

But our moment of levity did not last long when I asked, 'So do you think that CoviDEM will end up being more or less serious than regular ADEM problems?'

'We don't know,' he said. 'But given the devastation Covid inflicts on the lungs, more serious than other types of pneumonia, and what it does to the rest of the body, I fear it's almost certainly going to be worse.'

Oh God, I thought, *it's just like punch after punch in the stomach.* 'Well, we'll just have to keep hoping he is that exception,' I said weakly.

'I'm very, very sorry that this has happened to you,' he said. 'He has been exceptionally unlucky. What has happened is rare, and it is incredibly rare in adults. But we're going to see more of it, I fear, a lot more neurological problems. We already know Covid causes strokes and brain bleeds. But this kind of inflammatory effect is new. I'm afraid Derek is at the crest of a really grim wave.'

'Being an ICU patient, knowing you've nearly died or being told you've nearly died, must be terrifying,' I said. 'Surely there'll be post-traumatic stress disorder on a massive scale.'

He agreed.

Now more and more people who were never even hospitalized for Covid, who were considered mild cases, are weeks and months later reporting short-term memory loss, pains and loss of function in hands and feet, their fine motor skills affected, which is now being investigated as nerve damage. I met a nurse who was extremely successful before she contracted Covid – she was in charge of three wards. But even though she had never been taken into hospital, as her case wasn't considered severe at the time, months on she was barely able to function. She said she had lost all 'executive function', the bit of the brain that controls how you plan and make decisions. She couldn't even trust herself to make a meal: she would forget she had put a pan on and was worried she would burn the house down.

Talking to Dr L was helpful and I was grateful for his time, but it was so much to take in – I always thought of questions afterwards, or needed further explanation once the call had ended. Thanks to the ever-supportive Sir Elton John, we managed to track down neurologists and experts in America to supplement my information. My friend Carla Romano got hold of contacts in France and Italy and, step by step, I made a collection of opinions to fill out the bigger picture. There were no quick answers, no magic solutions, and they all seemed to say that time was what we had to cling to: time for the doctors to learn more, and time for Derek's body to heal. They confirmed that steroids and plasma exchange were the best options, although they were all frustrated and concerned that the treatment was coming so late in Derek's journey. That, coupled with precise twenty-four-hour expert care, to help all areas of his body heal, was the way forward. And I knew that that was what the wonderful health teams were giving. It reassured me that he was on the right path.

Speaking to other experts also gave me the chance to ask the questions I knew Derek's direct team wouldn't want to answer. With one neurologist in America I asked what happened if the steroids and plasma exchange didn't work: was there nothing beyond time and waiting? He said that, apart from hoping that his body healing could have a positive effect, there was 'brain plasticity'. For years, it had been thought the brain couldn't heal, but now they knew it could through 'plasticity' or, as he put it, 'rerouting'. He gave me the analogy of driving down a freeway and suddenly finding the road blocked because of an accident. Immediately your brain will try to find a route around the obstacle from your existing knowledge of the area and your experience. You will find an alternative road and head off on it quite happily, although maybe more slowly and your journey might take longer. That, he explained, is what the brain does, and what doctors do is try to trigger the brain to take the right alternative road with rehab. It felt good to know that the treatment Derek was getting wasn't the end of the story, that there might be more things to try.

'I know it sounds daft,' I asked, 'but do you think it makes any difference that Derek is clever?'

He laughed. 'Well, you won't get me on record saying this because the entire "woke" world would come down on me like a ton of bricks but, yes, it does in a way, though it's not as simple as having a big IQ. What we do think, though, is that the more *thinking* you've done in your life, the more things you've conquered, the more learning, brain training you've been through, the more pathways you've laid down and the more alternatives you have to access.'

At last Derek's colourful life, his dramas, his depression, his triumphs, his failures, his comebacks, might help him when he needed it most.

Beyond the monitoring of his treatment, I was also determined to try to communicate with Derek as much as I possibly could. The only way to get through was on the phone and I knew it tied up the staff's time. We needed a separate system.

Our first stumbling block was trying to get hold of an iPad for him, as at this point there were none in stock in the entire country. Apple was perpetually selling out and with most of the Western world home schooling, we weren't the only ones desperate to get our hands on an extra device. Eventually Ben Wegg-Prosser managed to get one from his office, and we set it up so that we had a system of codes. There was a code word that I would give the staff so they knew it was me when I rang, and we set up the device so that they could call me by pressing a single button. Just because you're a brilliant nurse or carer doesn't mean you'll have time to become a technology-minded iPad expert, after all. And I knew they were stretched to the limit with patients, coping with more every single day.

On the other hand, a few people with a public profile had now been seriously ill, which meant that hospitals needed some sort of security for calls, especially video calls. So we had a slightly silly but very reassuring situation where I would ring up and they would go, 'Oh hi, Kate.' And I would go, 'Hello. I'm just seeing if I can do a FaceTime with Derek, please,' and they'd go, 'Password, please,' with a smile.

Every time I rang, I was thinking, Right, what could trigger him? What anecdote might connect? Should I be trying to make him laugh, giving him a rallying pep talk? What would do the trick in getting through, helping him to know it's us, that we're here, that life is out there?

The steroid and plasma exchange courses lasted for two weeks, and we were monitoring closely for any sign of improvement. I would speak to the team every day, but progress was slow. Occasionally they would get a flicker of movement: a twitch of a thumb or a jerk of a foot. They put special electrical pads on Derek's feet to measure any kind of resistance, the tiniest flicker of muscle push. Sometimes it would register, sometimes not. And it was never clear whether it was an involuntary jerk, like when you're dreaming in a deep sleep, or intentional, a response that meant Derek was starting to wake up.

There were two FaceTime conversations when the nurses said to me, 'We think he can definitely hear. He jumps if a car backfires outside or if someone drops a metal tray of equipment, for example.' But could he interpret what he could hear? Or was it just a reflex reaction?

The nurses would hold the iPad close to his face. He couldn't move, but sometimes it would seem as though his eyes swivelled in my direction. Sometimes it seemed he was looking hard at me, really, *really* trying, and the team in the room would be saying, 'He's focusing on your voice, he's definitely focusing on your voice.'

But there was no proof that it wasn't just because a blue-lit oblong tablet was flickering in front of him, rather than that he knew my face or voice. So I asked them to put his glasses on – even before he was ill, his sight wasn't very good. I felt that helped, because maybe he had been looking at a blur. But we didn't know if he could see at all or if the Covid had caused him to lose his sight, as had happened in other patients. Tests showed his optic nerve was working but it wasn't clear what was being processed.

I felt that he was starting to focus on me. I started to record the video calls to show to close friends, to check that it wasn't just me over-investing in any small change. 'What do you think?' I asked, and one said immediately, 'Oh my God, that's so much better than the last time.' But it was hard to tell what was real progress and what wasn't.

It was a period that felt like months and months and months, but also as if everything was moving very quickly. It reminded me of those early days after having a baby, when you lose all sense of time. I remembered in my first days after leaving hospital saying confidently to my mum,

'Darcey doesn't usually sleep in the mornings.' My mum laughed. 'Darling, she's barely a week old. She doesn't have a "usually" yet!' But of course to me it had felt like a lifetime. Time was muddled in a similar way now, shifting like it does in an old episode of *Doctor Who*. Backwards and forwards it would go, one minute me saying, 'Oh, that was ages ago,' before realizing it had been three hours ago, not last week.

The spectre behind all of this was the constant fear that he was no longer there, that he had already gone. One thing that became clear to me during this period was how many of the expressions on our faces are unintentional, the little things that others see that make us *us* to them. When we look in the mirror, we see what we look like when we're happy, smiling, cross or frowning, and we think our loved ones use those expressions to judge how we're feeling. But actually they see myriad things in our faces all of the time. How we look when we're reading or watching TV, or struggling with a particularly tricky challenge – they dance across our faces while we're entirely oblivious. It's the unintentional expressions that make up the person we know. I had thought I'd be looking for Derek to be bursting into tears and saying, 'I love you, thank God you're here,' by now. Instead, I was looking for the micro-expressions that possibly only I could spot.

But the complete paralysis of his face had robbed Derek of even the chance of these little clues. He was either frozen lifeless or gave the twitches and jerks I occasionally spotted, which were so alien to the usual Derek that they made him seem less like himself, not more.

By now the two weeks it had taken to get the plasma exchange and the steroids into Derek's system had long passed. I was encouraged as they said it might take more weeks to show any result, but even so, those weeks had passed with no change. Teams came on and off Derek's shifts, saying, 'Let's see where he is when I'm back on duty', only to return to find little had progressed.

Eventually it was left to Dr W to call me with the inevitable verdict that the plasma exchange and steroids, though worth a try, had indeed been too little too late.

'Don't give up on him, please, Dr W,' I begged. 'I know he's still in there. Please keep trying.'

'God, no,' he said. 'No one is giving up, Kate, I promise you. This is where the real work begins. In fact, we know how hard these weeks have been and we think we've found a way that we can allow you to visit him.'

To see him, to touch him … Maybe, just maybe, if I held his hand he would know I was there and could squeeze it back. If he sensed I was there, maybe that would give us a miracle.

'You won't be able to touch him,' Dr W said, as if he had read my mind. 'It will have to be like a sort of prison visit, and you'll have to wear the full PPE, but it's a start and we think we can make that happen tomorrow. Are you free?'

Free! I would have cancelled the Queen to make that appointment! Of course I was free!

Darcey and Billy were so excited for me, even though they were disappointed that they couldn't go too. Billy constructed a Lego 'family' of figures with 'Dad in the centre as he is the most important' and the rest of us, including grandparents, on either side.

'Dad loved doing Lego with me. It will remind him and make him feel less lonely in the hospital on his own,' he explained.

Darcey sketched his portrait, comical but actually with a reasonable likeness. She also wrote him a long letter, saying he had to get better quickly as she was getting cleverer every day: if he didn't wake up soon, he would never win an argument with her ever again. Typical of their constant goading of each other. I felt almost giddy with excitement, blow-drying my hair and putting makeup on, picking out an outfit. It was as if Derek and I had a date, that the distance of the last few months was falling away.

I had longed for months to see him, but instead of the wonderful reunion of my imagination, it was a physical manifestation of everything we now faced together.

For so long, in so many dark moments, I had envisaged us rushing into each other's arms again. The tears, the intense eye-to-eye smiles, the reunion any of us might dream of. But what actually happened was so very different. And I was unprepared for it. I had not seen Derek since that time I had gone in to bring him a few things before he was put into his coma, months before. Even though I had been looking at him on the iPad, the nurses had always held it close, so I could see only his face, partly so I could try to connect to his eyes more but also maybe to spare me seeing how many tubes were going in and out of him, and everything he was hooked up to. Also, his beard had grown long, so its bushiness hid how thin his face was. I had got used to looking past the frozen reality of the state he was in, ignoring the paralysis and staring straight into his eyes, looking for life.

My mind was racing as I arrived at the hospital and waited while they made sure all safety precautions and isolation measures were in place.

Even now it remains hard for me to describe how I felt when I was led into the room. It was like a white ball of shock so bright you want to put your hand up to your eyes to protect them. In an instant, it became clear that the reality of his devastation had been only hypothetical to me until now. Fear reported to me by phone calls in a world where no one left their home any more; snatches of his face on a screen, in a world where everyone had to communicate digitally, all day. Unreal, intangible, unimaginable. And now the hypothetical had become physical, unmistakable, real.

Derek was unrecognizable. Legs like sticks, thinner than I'd thought his previously big frame could make possible. His arms too ... How could muscle, flesh and fat become something so small? Even his bones should be bigger than that, surely. His lungs heaved, mechanically wrenching in and out in an unnatural, desperate way. His eyes stared straight up as he lay on the bed, which I was grateful for as I didn't want him to see my reaction. How could I bring comfort to him, tell him he was going to be OK, when he was in this state?

I thought I would faint. 'Can I have a chair, please?' I said limply.

Someone brought one into the room, meticulously wiping it down and covering it with disposable sheets. I sat down, realizing I was an alien, a danger, no help to Derek at all. Even being there meant they had to clean afterwards, disinfect my presence away.

I rallied. It wasn't possible for him to know I was there … I needed to give him the connection, something to hold on to, a rope he could catch somewhere deep inside so that I could haul him out.

I stood up. 'Is there any way he could see me? Can I get any closer to him?'

I wasn't allowed to, but they managed to angle the bed and raise it up enough until I could fix myself in his eyeline.

'Derek, it's Kate,' I said. 'I'm here. I'm always here. You're safe in a hospital where they're going to get you better.'

I was almost shouting this now, as if turning up the volume would somehow bridge the divide. I looked deep into his eyes and said, 'I know you can't respond, you're too weak and sick, but I know you're in there. I know you love us and we all love you. I am going to get you out, though. Don't be worried. I'm here.'

When I said 'out', I meant out of being trapped inside himself, but also out of the hospital, home, safe. I wanted him to believe that I knew he was in there while he was spending days being prodded and tested by strangers. I wanted him to feel he didn't have to prove anything to me, that someone understood he was still present – even though I was far from sure. I pulled my mask down, which I wasn't supposed to do but I wanted him to see my face. His eyes were fixed on me, but with no movement in the surrounding muscles they looked blank.

'I know you're still in there. Derek, I continue to know that you love us. We all love you. And I'm going to get you out. I'm going to do it. We're going to do it together, just like we always do everything together, and you're going to be OK.'

Then my time was up. I was whisked away.

I have no memory of leaving the hospital or getting into the taxi home. My phone kept ringing: Derek's mum and my parents. I couldn't collect myself enough to answer, I was sobbing uncontrollably, sobbing and shaking. But I couldn't go home. I couldn't hide this level of shock and distress from the children. There was no way of masking it. But they had never seen me like this and it would be horrific for them.

I got out two streets from my home to gather myself, to delay the inevitable. Derek's sister Sue called, and I was relieved, thinking she would know best what to tell her mum and what to keep from her. I could no longer judge.

I was hyperventilating, saying, 'He's bad, he's really, really bad. You know, he's not moving. He's completely paralysed, like, he can't move even the muscles of his face. He's changed for ever. Please, you have to help me. I can't do this. I'm scared for the children. I need someone to come. Do you think you or Di could drive your mum and dad down? They could sit in the garden with the children. They needn't go near me. I just need to lock myself in my room and cry for thirteen or fourteen hours, to process this, to get a grip on myself.'

She started sobbing and I realized she was in shock too. I knew it was unfair to burden her but I couldn't stop crying.

'It's not for me, it's for the children … I have to get control of myself. I'm scared if they see me like this …' I tried to explain.

She couldn't come, of course. No one could. Her parents were too vulnerable to take the risk. She had her own children, and she was dealing with her own shock, as each of us was.

Oh God, I thought, the cavalry isn't coming. No one can help. The doctors don't know what's going on. My visit hasn't waved a wand and cast a spell. Derek hasn't miraculously woken up. No one can help. I am alone and drowning.

Then I seemed to snap to. I realized how unfair I was being. 'Don't worry, Sue. I'll think of something. It'll be OK. I'll talk to you later.'

But nothing came to mind. I carried on walking, then called Rob Rinder. I just poured it all out, hours of pain, of crying, of fear. I was sitting on the kerb, sobbing into the gutter, and he listened in his usual practical way.

'Right, stop thinking,' he said. 'And that's an order. You're in medical shock. There's nothing you can do right now but sleep. Go home, then go upstairs, close your eyes and sleep. That is your one task.'

The simplicity seemed to work. Making it a medical problem that I couldn't fix, rather than my failure to cope, somehow shifted things. I went home, putting a smile on my face, and opened the door, somehow managing to say, 'Yes, Dad loved all your things. He's weak but doing well. Now let's watch some telly, whatever you want, because I think I'm just going to fall asleep.'

It worked.

The next day my dad rang. There were more tears, but he said something so simple that it really helped me over the following weeks and months. 'You know it's going to be two years before the doctors really feel there's nothing more they can do, if he hasn't changed from the state he's in now. So stop fast-forwarding to that point: take it one day at a time. You have no idea how you'll feel when that point comes. You have no idea where Derek will be by that time. You haven't got the information to form that picture yet so stop trying. It's just as likely things will be fine as not. There is no evidence of otherwise, so hang on to that hope and don't speculate.'

The children seemed happy, playing their games outside, and I functioned enough to keep going, although I could no longer wrestle any joy from watching them leap about. 'Be careful, you might get hurt,' I fretted. I couldn't be carefree. It was impossible to delude myself that they wouldn't get hurt, that the worst wouldn't happen, because it was so bad for Derek.

'Mum, you're turning into Dad,' Darcey said. 'He used to be the worrier and now you are too.'

She knew something was wrong, something had changed. I would catch her looking at me, worried, until I turned and plastered the smile back on my face. Then one day, seemingly from nowhere, she suddenly asked, 'Mum, are you going to kill yourself?'

I literally jumped, like I'd been startled by a knock at the door. 'No! What do you mean? What on earth would make you say that?'

'Because you're so sad all the time about Dad.'

'No, absolutely not, Darcey. It couldn't be any more the opposite of that. I've never wanted to live more. I'm not going to kill myself. No. I *hate* the idea you've been thinking that, worrying about it,' I said.

'Well, I haven't *really*, I just thought it was best to check, to say it out loud.'

This was classic Darcey. Maybe she was more like me than I realized. Face the worst, then anything else seems easier.

'I'm not worried about Dad,' she went on. 'Yeah, I think he's gonna be fine. I've manifested it. I've said in my head, "Dad's gonna be fine." And he will, whatever way. He's got doctors looking after him. But I'm worried about how you are on your own.'

'I'm really sorry. I don't want you to worry about me. That's the exact opposite of what I want. I want you not to be worried about me. And I'm not on my own – I have you and Bill, lots of friends and family, and we're all going to get through this together. I know how much you miss Dad and I want to protect you from worrying.'

'Well, stop trying so hard, because you're very bad at hiding when you're worried.'

'OK,' I said. 'When I'm sad, I'll just say, "I need to be on my own," and we'll work out a plan so we can get through. I can't promise you that Dad will be exactly the same. And I can't even really promise you that he's going to get a hundred per cent better. I believe he is and the doctors believe he's doing better and better. But I can promise you that I'm not going to kill myself. That is a cast-iron promise.'

Darcey nodded. 'Good. That's sorted, then. Now, while we're talking, I have one more question.'

God, what could it be? I dreaded to hear what she was going to say.

'Mum, can I have a dog?'

And we were back! She knew she was pushing it, and we both collapsed into fits of giggles. We were going to be OK.

Chapter 9

The New Normal

My daughter's question, 'Are you going to kill yourself?' had spun me on my axis.

Yes, I knew she liked to shock, to put into words what others avoid saying out of fear, embarrassment or concern about its effect on others. Darcey sees those constraints and runs straight at them, just like Derek. So I knew she wasn't in the dark mental place that other teenagers might have been had they asked that. But, still, it brought me up sharp.

I had to make changes. We had been in a bubble of three, and I had been torn between that bubble and 'Project Save Derek', dividing myself between making them feel nothing but safety, and facing total lack of safety where Derek was concerned. I had been trying to absorb all my fears and not inflict them on Billy and Darcey, so they could feel Dad's absence was temporary. I thought I'd been keeping aloft

211

the idea that he could still walk through the door, saying, 'Where's my dinner?' and life could pick up again.

I never wavered in the hope that Derek could come back to us, but it was now clear it wasn't going to be a magical wake-up, an instant, miraculous reversion to the life we'd had before. Derek would be changed, even if it was 'just' emotionally, as a result of the trauma of a near-death experience. And we were becoming changed by all this too.

I had to break out of the bubble, to try to get on with life. How we had been living wasn't healthy for the children. It was bad enough that they didn't have their dad: I couldn't let them think that their lives and our future had been swept away, too, when he'd got into the ambulance. If I couldn't return us to the old normal right now, I had to create a new normal, a way for *us* to exist, for our lives to go on while we were 'waiting for Dad'.

But I felt guilty. I had been living with one focus, the crisis, for so long that it felt as if making any plans for a future before Derek was home was somehow giving up on him, loosening my hold on the hope that he would return.

'I know I have to take life off pause somehow, for Darcey and Billy's sake, but it feels wrong,' I explained to my friend Clare. 'I feel guilty, as if I'm deserting Derek. I worry that if I take my attention away from him for an instant, it's like taking my eye off the ball. What if something is missed?'

'Rubbish,' she said. 'It's exactly what Derek would want you to do. You have to keep a life for him to go back to and you can't stay in this focused tiny world, or it will consume you. And that's not helping anyone.'

'But what about your beloved manifesting? Your idea of keeping your focus on what you want so it feeds out to the universe?' I asked. Manifesting had been one of the ways Clare and Vickie had helped me to overcome my fear, and my sense of helplessness. It was one of the ways I tried to make hope *real*. If I stopped keeping that image focused, at the forefront of my mind, wasn't I allowing it to fade? Maybe – gulp – risking it disappearing?

'Aagh,' she said. 'I think you're ready for next-level manifesting. Manifesting when done properly is about taking off the pressure of focusing. You fix on what you want, but not as a wish. You make it concrete, and part of that is just having it there as a core belief. You believe the world is round, don't you? You don't need to keep looking it up in a book, constantly circumnavigating the globe to know it's round. You just know it and you get on with life accordingly. You just have to *know* that Derek is going to get better, believe that hope is real, and get on with life. It's not letting hope go. To my way of thinking, it's making hope *more* real.'

'O-K ...' I said, somewhat doubtfully.

She then went on to tell me a story, to give me a new mental picture.

'Imagine living in a town which is perfect. Everyone's happy, everyone's employed, the air is clean. It's a wonderful community. You arrived as a stranger to the town. You're thinking, This is absolutely great. I love this! And you settle in and start living there, carefree, feeling you've arrived at last. Then someone says to you, "Oh, by the way, be careful, I heard there's a big pothole in the town centre. It might cause an accident." Then, every time you drive down that high street, you're nervous about the pothole. You're looking out for it. You aren't even sure it's there, it might just be a rumour, but now, because of this warning, you're staying alert, looking for it just in case it catches you out. Now it's on your mind all the time. It starts to dominate things for you. You no longer notice the pretty buildings, the friendly people, the clean air. You don't even enjoy driving through the place. The perfect town becomes unliveable for you, for as long as that's what you're focusing on. Where is the pothole? And what trouble might it cause?'

I got it. Everything the doctors and neurologists were saying was focusing me on the pothole, not on the expanse of land around it. It wasn't their fault. They had to warn me appropriately. But I had to put these warnings into perspective. I had to take my mind away from the pothole because we didn't *know* if it even existed. We didn't know if the pothole was going to kill Derek, or me, or damage us, or if someone could repair it before it became a disaster. We also didn't know whether, if we *did* encounter the pothole, we'd be able to navigate around it.

She was telling me to look about, to focus on what was good, to be grateful, not guilty, and move forward.

'Don't get lost in fear and the negative,' she said. 'Get some perspective and help the children to get some too.'

It helped me start to plan how to create some kind of new normal in a world that was just waking up. I was aware that lockdown was lifting, restrictions lightening. People were starting to rediscover each other and the world around them. Shops were opening; workers were returning to their offices; bars and restaurants were raising their shutters and serving customers in every spot of outdoor space that they could find.

We were like moles, creeping out blinking into the light and loving it, despite our fears. Even though there was sadness in knowing that Derek couldn't move on with us, I was also painfully aware that, unlike so many others, he was still alive. It was wonderful to see everyone starting to gain confidence in themselves and their neighbourhoods all over again, and I wanted Darcey and Billy to be a part of that too – despite Derek's situation.

On my brother Matthew's advice, we decided to start small, to venture out a bit at a time.

'Come on,' I said. 'Let's go out.'

The kids were nervous, particularly Billy. Having been told to stay at home for so long, they were fearful of catching the thing that had taken their dad from them. I suggested we start with a drive, just to get the lie of the land. It was strange seeing other people, and the shops opening. Billy's favourite toy shop had closed down, a victim of lockdown. It was one of those old-style toy shops that had a table of bits and bobs, yo-yos, finger puppets and mini Slinkys at pocket-money prices. We had often gone there after school on a Friday, ever since he was little, as a start to the weekend. 'Oh, no!' he cried, visibly upset as we drove past its boarded-up windows. It was as if a part of his childhood had closed down too, and I sensed his loss.

'Bill, we'll make new memories,' I promised him.

On that first trip round the neighbourhood, neither of them wanted to get out of the car. But it was a start. It helped Billy and Darcey to see that others had been affected, to see that job losses and livelihoods were being grieved everywhere, that it wasn't just our family.

I wanted to get back into our community. I remembered how wonderful it had been to be part of Clap for Carers, to feel that sense of coming together. But it had been painful when it came to an end – I sensed other people breathe a sigh of relief that the 'crisis was over', but we still felt locked in ours. Now it was time to reach out and connect again.

I joined the local WhatsApp groups, and the first notification I saw was that someone in our road had cleared out their shed during lockdown and had three old bikes they wanted to get rid of. 'Our children left home ten years ago so these will definitely need a service but they're welcome to anyone who wants them,' said the message. It felt as if Fate was pushing us to get out there.

We went to collect them and it was so wonderful to meet new people on our road. They were so kind in helping us get the bikes up and running, and we had a giggle when Darcey and Billy picked the best two (obviously), leaving me with the one that looked as though it was for a nine-year-old. I tried to pedal with my knees under my chin.

We started going for short rides in the evening, just to the local playground (masks on and keeping our distance from others), until we felt a little braver. It got us out into the world, seeing others walking dogs and playing. One evening, a family walked past us, laughing, the dad carrying a child on his shoulders, just as Derek had done with Darcey and Billy when they were younger.

Darcey stared at them as they passed and I knew she was thinking about her dad. 'Mum, can I ask you something?'

I braced myself.

'Are we ever going on holiday again?'

Her mind had seen his absence, raced backwards to all the things we loved doing together and then wondered how they would work now on a practical level.

'Yes, absolutely, of *course* we are,' I said. 'Mind you, no one is really travelling at the moment. Are you wondering whether we'll be going away, the three of us, and how that will work with Dad?'

I felt she was thinking about the future, not just about the sadness of him being away from us, but how we could make things work if he didn't return to how he was.

'Yes,' she said. 'I was thinking we could still go away on planes, because I've seen people on the news travelling with tubes in them. But I think we should start going first class as there'll definitely be more room there for a stretcher or a wheelchair.'

So practical and yet so impractical at the same time.

'Well, it's certainly a good thought,' I said, not wanting to crush her. 'But of course there's expense in that.'

'I've been thinking about that too. I think you should allow me to run Dad's company until he gets better. And you should go back to work too. They say the schools are going to open up soon so you won't need to look after us. Someone has to start earning money.'

She was right. Derek's company *was* Derek, so it hadn't earned a bean since he got sick. My bosses at Global and ITV had found ways to support me but I couldn't rely on their generosity for ever. This was a long-term situation we were dealing with, and it was going to take more than belief to keep me and the kids going. Not just fed and clothed, but keeping the children safe in the knowledge that their mum wasn't going to disappear on them too. We couldn't carry on like this indefinitely.

The cavalry wasn't coming, I reminded myself again. It was all down to me. Well, me, with some heroic friends and family.

By this time, we were allowed to have visitors in the garden, and one of the first people to come round was my friend Vickie. 'We need to open your post. And we need to work out your finances,' she told me.

I was panic-stricken.

'I know you haven't read any of it and I know you haven't done anything about it,' she said, as only an old friend could. 'Let me go through it with you, because I'm worried about your money. I'm here to be practical, to do what you can't. I'm going to sit with you, we're going to call your bank, and we're going to sort it all out.'

And we did. Well, at least we made a start on it. I *had* been worried about it all. I knew I was luckier than a lot of people because I had supportive bosses and a good job that was being kept open for me, but I also knew that, in those envelopes, trouble was brewing.

Every time I had tried to sort out any financial admin I had been stymied, either by a fresh crisis or because our accounts were solely in Derek's name or in both of our names so I couldn't access them on my own. They were locked. Because he was still technically in a coma, but not in a vegetative coma, it was a strange in-between world in terms of getting access to the accounts. On top of that, I couldn't find any life insurance for Derek – because, it transpired, he didn't have any. I couldn't find any critical health insurance either, which I was sure he had. It turned out that he was in the process of transferring everything over from one company to another when he got sick and went into hospital. On his phone I found a heartbreaking email, which had come in just after he went into hospital, saying everything was ready for him to sign. But of course he had never had the chance.

It felt good to conquer the emotional block of opening Derek's post, trying to unravel the mysteries with Vickie's help. At least the sorting had begun.

Not long after this I had a phone call from a friend, who started the conversation by saying, 'Now, listen, Kate, we'll never talk about this again, but someone did this for me when I lost my husband and I was a freelancer. The least I can do is to organize it for someone else.'

I had no idea what she was talking about but she continued, 'A group of my friends got together and decided that each of them would give whatever they could afford, then one person transferred the money to me. Some of us have done the same for you. I'll transfer the money and then we never have to talk about it again, because none of us doubts that you'll get back on your feet before long.'

'I don't even know what account you could transfer it into,' I explained. 'They're all locked because Derek and I had a company together. I don't have power of attorney because he's alive.'

In the end I found a card for an account I'd had when I was a student, the last account that had been solely in my name and pre-dated Derek. I reactivated it and my friends put money into it. They repeated that we never had to talk about it again, but I hope one day to pay them back.

It was an amazing thing to do. I was so overwhelmed with gratitude, and so aware of how lucky I was in so many ways. To some degree, the incredible kindness of everyone around me made me feel a little guilty that I still wasn't functioning properly. I couldn't have asked any more of people because they had given so much, emotionally and practically, and so many were sick or had been sick themselves.

I just *have* to come back from this, I found myself thinking, because I can't *just* be grateful any more. At first, it left me shaky, to be the recipient of so much good luck amid so much bad, but in the end it galvanized me to head back into the world, and try to make the best of it.

Something else was pushing us back into the world: Billy's school was allowing year-six pupils to return. I was so pleased for him – he absolutely deserved to get back to his friends and his life while all of this horror was going on with Derek. But it left me with a lump in my throat that he was passing through huge life stages without his dad by his side.

There are all the little things that every year-six child

goes through, but last year was different from any other. Normally, there's so much to mark the end of term. At Billy's school in year six there was always a camping trip, and stories of the adventure get passed down year after year. This time, it was cancelled. The end-of-year show was cancelled too. Billy had been hoping to be the Artful Dodger in *Oliver!* – he'd already been practising the songs when Derek got sick. Missing the show obviously wasn't comparable to missing his dad, but it was a reminder, yet another, that things were so far from our expectations of just a couple of months ago.

He loved being back at school but the end-of-term assembly was traumatic. It was, of course, a Zoom event, with the kids in the school hall and the parents watching at home on their laptops. The school and the kids had put so much effort into making it celebratory, and inclusive. There was such a huge collective sigh of relief that we had all made it to the end of term, and I was so proud of Billy for all he'd achieved. Then they played a compilation video of some of the great times the children had had while they were at the school, one moment of which included some footage of Derek on a school trip. He was always the first to volunteer for such things – he adored them. And the kids loved having him there. But we had no forewarning we might catch a glimpse of him on the screen. The children hadn't seen him at all since March, and no one had heard that big booming voice and certainly not seen him as he had been. Suddenly he was there, playing, laughing, full of mischief, full of life. It was heartbreaking, blindsiding, especially as Billy was there in the hall and I couldn't give him the hug I was so sure he desperately needed.

Straight after the assembly I was due to visit Derek at the hospital. I'd been looking forward to it for weeks. But I sat in his hospital room, looking at the difference between the man I had seen on the screen an hour earlier and the man beside me now, and just cried and cried. Derek would have walked over hot coals and broken glass to get to that assembly. And there he was, trapped by the damage of Covid, immobile, just lying there and staring. I didn't even know if he remembered who Billy was. We still had no evidence that he remembered anything of me, us, or his life before.

I couldn't carry on waiting for change. I had to start working. Apart from anything else, Derek had to have a life to come back to and I needed to maintain a family life that functioned.

The first thing to do was talk to my bosses about giving an interview. There was so much to consider. I didn't feel as if I could just pop up on air and not say anything about what we'd been through when there had been a fair amount of media around Derek being so ill. Also, knowing Derek's personality, I felt sure he would have wanted to tell his own story. I felt a huge responsibility to him and, of course, to his family.

But I also knew that in Derek's work, both in politics and in his psychology, that if nothing else, he would be comforted that he was helping others who came after him. And this was true. The doctors *had* changed treatment pathways as his recovery progressed. I thought he would like the idea, even if he never did come back, that he had been helpful.

It was agreed that I would go on to *Good Morning Britain* on the Friday morning, not as a host but as an interviewee, and afterwards I would speak to lovely Jane Moore, whom I've known for years, and who is on *Loose Women* but also works for the *Sun*. Up until this point, I had been in our bubble with the children and only one or two visitors. I had seen Derek and I had seen those caring for him, and started to venture out into the world, saying hi across the street to neighbours and watching strangers on our cycle rides. But I had seen nothing else from my life before, nothing of my old routine, nothing of how I even used to present myself. For two decades it had been a life of working in a newsroom, and one of the great perks of being an onscreen host is getting my hair blow-dried and makeup put on for me before I have to face the world. That, of course, wouldn't be happening at the moment.

It had been months of unshaven legs and wearing my plastic gardening clogs pretty much every day. Those clogs had been a Christmas gift to me from my parents, instantly becoming a joke between Darcey and me. When I'd opened them I'd looked at her and thought, Oh my gosh, I'll never wear those ... but I'd barely taken them off because they were so comfortable.

Suffice to say, glamour-wise, I was in a state. The thought of going back in front of a camera gave me the feeling you used to get when you went back to school after the summer and the uniform felt rough and scratchy. Your body had forgotten how to be that you, after a summer of near *Swallows and Amazons* freedom, and suddenly you had to step back into it all. I felt as if I were shifting between worlds.

And, like the rest of us, with the hairdressers closed, my hair was almost beyond help. On Instagram many people were cutting each other's hair and painting their roots, going for ginger, pink, blue hair, the works. But that was not for me. Instead, the night before the interview, Darcey said, 'I'll do your hair. I can cut it.' My first response was, 'Umm, I'm not sure that's a good idea.' But what were the other options? So, that evening Darcey sat down and cut my hair. It was so sweet, because one of the things that was trending on Twitter the next day was #Darceysbob!

We had a full-on hairdressing session. I did Billy's, Darcey did mine, and neither of us was allowed to touch hers. She could get away with it as she's got lovely long straight hair, and it just looked a bit long – if Billy's goes beyond six weeks without a cut, he looks like the child of Albert Einstein and Boris Johnson. And he was so far past six weeks that he had gone past Boris Johnson and turned into some kind of surf dude. I just looked like a mad hermit who lived in a cave. Perhaps an old crone who lived in the woods, whom the younger folk of the village might go to for herbal advice. All in all, it was a good job Darcey stepped up. It was almost as if she was saying, 'Let me help you to be ready to go back.'

We even had a session when Darcey waxed my legs. It was absolutely murderous – she loved it! Around this time she had been doing a much better job than I was of taking control of her environment. She had been designing things for her bedroom, and making the flatpack furniture we had bought for her in the pre-Covid spring, while on FaceTime to her dad. She would just sit there, talking him through what she was doing, where she was planning to put it, what her design vision was. And now she was getting me ready to go back to work.

I had been thinking I didn't know how to prepare for the interview because I'm a woman of facts, as you now know. I take copious notes, colleagues always laughing at me, saying, 'When are you ever going to need that?' It's because it helps me to order my thoughts. At home I had box files full of notes, but I also knew that it wasn't the detail of Derek's blood-oxygen levels that I needed to get across in the interview, so there was little I could do to prepare, beyond Darcey's beauty salon.

The interview had to be in our garden, for Covid safety and insurance reasons. I would be at home, and Ben Shephard in the studio. They sent over a producer I'd worked with for twenty years, and when he arrived that morning, I felt as if I was seeing a traveller from a different era. It was as if he and the crew had arrived from another world, one I had forgotten about and missed sorely. Of course, they had all been going through hell themselves, with all sorts of professional and personal changes, but the producer seemed the same. When I walked into the back garden with him, I felt weirdly as if I was in a dream, that all of the months that had gone before ... were they even real? It was like a flashback. Dipping a toe into a previous life and realizing it had still been there all along. I had craved it, been desperate for it, yet it didn't seem real at all.

I was so nervous about the interview, mainly because I felt an enormous sense of responsibility. I didn't want to scare people. I wanted to do right by Derek, by his family, and by all of the doctors and nurses who had been working so hard for so long.

ITV asked if there was anywhere I didn't want them to go with this interview and I said, 'Not really. I'm just going to say what I feel Derek would feel comfortable with me saying, which is also the truth, that this has devastated every part of his body. Every organ is damaged.'

I also felt I had a duty to share our story, because I wanted people to know, most importantly, that Covid wasn't going away. *Even if you recover, the risk is huge*, I wanted to say. *Don't take it lightly, because people lost their lives*. The big point I wanted to make was: *Don't think this is a touch of flu. Some have died, some have recovered, but there are thousands more who are paying long-term costs even if they have survived. It can devastate your life for ever, even if you live*. The interview also gave me the opportunity to thank people for the love, the messages and the hope. I wanted to make sure I shared the reality of the situation without scaring anyone to death.

The interview was meant to last for fifteen minutes, but it ended up eating into the whole show, and lasting the best part of an hour. I have very little recollection of it. Normally, every time I come off air, the people I work with know that I instantly go into an absolute turmoil of scrutiny, thinking,

Oh, it's so frustrating that we didn't have more time with that guest because I wanted to ask them this; It's so frustrating that that happened; Why didn't I think of this? Basically, a constant wish to do things better.

Over the last twenty years, I've shared enormous amounts of my life. The people who watch ITV at breakfast time have known me since I first started, when I was married to someone else. Then I was divorced. Then there were the dating years and the craziness and the parties, meeting Derek and getting married to him. And then they saw me as I sat on the sofa every morning getting bigger and bigger when I was pregnant with Darcey. Then I came back with a little baby to share with them, and the same with Billy. I still get messages from people saying, 'Oh, I can't believe it. My daughter is eight now so yours must be this age too. I can remember while I was pregnant watching you with Darcey,' and it's an incredible bond. It's a huge honour to have been waking up with these people, being in people's bedrooms and front rooms for that amount of time and to have shared so much of my life with them, then have them share theirs with me just when I needed it.

It's one of the wonderful things about breakfast television: you're in people's homes just when they're at their most vulnerable, waking up, getting dressed, putting on mascara. It binds you and connects you. But to actually stand there and talk about probably the most devastating thing in my life, and the most devastating thing for the world, affecting an entire generation, felt like an overwhelming responsibility. For the first time ever, I talked without notes. I just talked and then did the same thing with James O'Brien on LBC, Global Radio. My being so open created the most enormous ripples. People reacted so kindly. Truly, it was wonderful.

Dr Hilary had helped to reinforce my message: 'What Kate is saying is so useful. She can help people to understand what all the experts and politicians can't or maybe don't even realize yet. People need to know that Covid isn't binary. Yes, we've been fighting a disease where you either live or die. But it's not just that. It can leave devastation that changes lives, too.'

By now it was June, the point at which everybody just wanted to get back to normal. There was a sense that we were on the downhill slope. The common mood seemed to be, 'I've had enough. It's so good to be out. I want to get back to work now.' We had stopped Clapping for Carers, and we had heard Dominic Cummings's tales of eye tests and seen Boris forgive him and move on. So, someone appearing and explaining that things might be a little more complicated than that created a bit of a stir, and I was horribly worried that I would just be making people miserable all over again.

The following day, the interview with Jane Moore filled the first six or seven pages of the *Sun*, and was on the cover of every newspaper. She did a great job, and she was as sensitive as she could be but there was no denying it was emotional to read, seeing the devastation in black and white, the true extent of how Covid had ripped through Derek's body.

I didn't dare go out to get the newspapers that morning. There were lots of photographers outside. Instead, I got someone to drop them off for me. It was a strange feeling, to see news about new leads in the Madeleine McCann story as a banner headline in the *Sun*, but me all over the front page. The headline was that Derek might never come out of the coma and there was a picture of me looking upset alongside it. As a journalist who has covered big stories and always tried to stick to the facts and handle them sensitively, it was very strange to be the subject of the headlines. I was trying not to be a scaremonger, or to shy away from the ugliness of the situation, but wanted to deliver my message with passion. I didn't feel remotely upset or angry with the *Sun* or any of the papers: I thought they did a wonderfully considerate job. But the reality was that it was uncomfortable to be both subject and journalist.

My editor told me that the segment of the show in which I was speaking was the first time that *Good Morning Britain* had beaten BBC *Breakfast* in the ratings, and they had done it by coming back to me over ad break after ad break to cover my family's story as sensitively as they possibly could. They were very happy from a professional point of view, but I also think they were right to do it, because they tapped into something no one else had: that a lot of people felt forgotten.

People had been through so much, and were starting to return to some semblance of normality, worrying about other things, even planning holidays. But *so many* people were feeling left behind and lost, whether because they were dealing with cancer and other diseases or because they were shielding and simply felt ignored. There was a feeling that one generation was going out and partying, celebrating like it was VE Day all over again, while another was trapped in bunkers all over the country.

This all meant that going back to work on air felt like a huge decision, as it might have been so fraught with repercussions. It was absolutely the right decision for me, for Derek, for the family. I'm glad that ITV and Global made it possible and were supportive – but the considerations on both sides were huge.

They were concerned about whether I would fall apart, whether it would be too much strain, whether I would be able to do the job at all. And there was another important point: the matter of silliness. The *Good Morning Britain* set-up has always been about tackling the biggest story of the day at one minute, and laughing about a viral video or a pop star who has done something ridiculous at the next. It's about silly fun over your cornflakes, us laughing at ourselves and each other, with the audience. And I think they just wondered how the audience would cope with that.

Would they see me as heartless, laughing and joking on air while my husband was still in hospital? Or would it look as if ITV were in some way exploiting me? Was it going to upset the viewers? Would it make them think I was exploiting *them* to be back at work talking about my story?

Then I realized that if I had been a nurse in a similar situation, I would have had to go back to work. Otherwise we'd all be in a mess. The whole country was trying to pick themselves up and get back to work. I wanted to do my part too. Plus, I had to send a signal to my children, and to myself, that life was going on, that it hadn't ended with Derek's diagnosis. The viewers, and my children, needed to know that they could be happy, and silly, and that no one would judge them for it after several incredibly difficult months. That was the sense of normal we were all craving.

Again, a guiding part of my decision-making was Derek himself. One of the things he always did, which used to drive me absolutely mad, was to stop and find the daftness in a crisis situation. Once, when Darcey was tiny, we nearly missed a flight home. We were coming back from Sicily, and we got to the airport too late – it was one of those flights where they overbook and you have to check in by a certain time or they give your seat away. And Derek was just being such an idiot about it, larking around and making Darcey laugh while I was freaking out that I was going to lose my job.

'I've got to get back! I've got to go to work!' I was hissing through my teeth. 'I'm on air tomorrow morning!'

But he just told me, 'You have to defuse the crises of life with laughter and silliness. It's the only way,' and he quoted Charlie Chaplin, who said that the best way to deal with pain is with humour.

We were certainly starting to see elements of this at home, where our descents into hysterical giggles were becoming more frequent as we found our feet in this new world. One afternoon while I was preparing to go back to work, Darcey had obviously been googling comas, now that we knew Derek was taking a long time to wake up. She came to me with a very serious face and said, 'Mum, I've been looking at comas on the internet, and when some people wake up, they have a completely different accent. One woman woke up and she was speaking Mandarin because she'd heard her nurse speaking it. She had just picked it up.'

'Oh, wow,' I said, worried about how worried she might be.

'What happens if Dad wakes up and he hasn't got a Chorley accent any more?' she said.

'What if he wakes up and sounds like Prince Charles?' I replied. We both burst into fits of giggles at the idea of our Chorley lad sounding like His Majesty.

It was such a break in tension, and as a result we felt very close to each other. She came and sat on my lap and we were laughing with tears in our eyes, which fourteen-year-olds don't often do. Then I looked at Billy, who was crying: 'I want Dad to still have his same accent ...'

'We're just laughing, Billy,' I tried to reassure him. 'It's funny ... Go on, do an impression of Dad talking like Prince Charles.' Billy is known in the family for doing the best impressions of Derek.

'Kay-ta, Kay-ta, I need my gribbins,' he started, remembering that Derek always called food 'gribbins' when he was being especially northern. He then did it as Prince Charles might have done. We were laughing and I just thought, This is so silly, and it's exactly what we need. And, actually, I think it's what everybody needs in a real crisis – to be able to have fun and laughter and joy.

So I trusted that the viewers of *Good Morning Britain*, and later the listeners of Smooth, would get it. And, actually, the reaction was the opposite of what senior management in both companies might have feared: people were so welcoming, a bit wobbly and nervous, but they thought, OK, you're real. You're not a presenter on a pedestal who leads a perfect life. You're a mum coming back to work like any de facto single mother.

I'm not a single mother really because Derek is still alive and here. But suddenly I had a lot of the practical considerations that single parents do. I was used to getting up at a quarter past two in the morning, knowing that someone was there taking care of the kids and making sure they got to school on time and in one piece. Now, I had to think about how I could get someone to make sure the children were safe and still be within the rules. It was a lot of logistical planning but only something that all single mothers have to do every day.

My first show back at *Good Morning Britain* was hugely emotional because whenever someone saw me their eyes would fill with tears. There was also a wall of affection, which was overwhelming in a wonderful way for me, but also overwhelming for everyone else. There were so many stories from viewers of what they'd been through and how they had got sick. I went on air and got through the show, held together by the viewers.

Afterwards, I experienced a strange feeling. As the adrenalin slipped away, my sense of achievement gave way to the realization that nothing had changed. Derek was still trapped. The first thing I wanted to do as soon as I came off air was to call him and say, 'Yes! It went OK!' The professional part of me that hadn't been able to do my job for all this time wanted that moment of celebration – but I couldn't share it with the one person I most wanted to. Instead I went into the dressing room and cried, thinking,

Oh, Derek, I just want you to be here now. And this hasn't changed anything. Being back on air wasn't a hurdle I had to get over that meant everything would now be OK. Of course it wasn't. It was just a first step.

I went to see him straight afterwards, to try to transfer to him some of the positive energy from the viewers.

It was not long after this that Derek started to move his right hand. It was the height of summer and there was a real sense that time was passing and the world was opening up. The team at the hospital said they didn't know for sure that he was purposefully moving his hand, but they thought sometimes he was. So on FaceTime I was saying all of my usual things to him: 'Darling, I know you're in there, I'm going to get you out. You're safe. The people around you are wearing masks because of Covid. You were very sick, but you're now getting better.'

And the team asked me to ask him to move his right hand. So I did. No response. Then they said, 'Ask him again, but this time leave a gap.' So I asked him again. And this time, he looked me really hard in the eye and moved his right hand. I wanted to burst with excitement. That was the first time there'd been any connection between us. They said it might have been incidental, but I was *sure* it wasn't.

I went in to see him again that week. And there was less shock, these days, about the change in him. I felt he was better, that he was brighter in the eyes. And I disagreed with Dr W that the plasma exchange and the steroids had made no difference. As if in confirmation, the team told me he was getting more movement in his tongue. Not the face but the tongue. So I said to him, 'Derek, stick your tongue out.' There was nearly a minute's delay, and I sat quietly watching him. Then … he stuck out his tongue.

I started to cry and cry. I was so proud! But, again, the team weren't sure. It felt as though they were constantly focusing on the negative, and I wanted now to physically push that away, thinking, It's not helpful. It's not a lack of belief that gets me through each day. Or a lack of hope.

Chapter 10

Anger and Despair

I was flipping backwards and forwards between two worlds, adjusting to two new normals. I was a single mum 'for the time being'; I always added that extra bit. While Derek is alive, he is just waiting to rejoin us.

I had another life too, though, one that was filled with doctors and nurses, late-night phone calls and constant research. And I was always asking: where might I find the magic pill that would bring Derek back?

I spent hours and hours talking to Derek on FaceTime. If there was a chance he could hear me I wanted him to know I was there. I wanted him to have something to focus on in his trapped state, locked in a prison of Covid damage, surrounded by well-meaning but unfamiliar voices, the alien bleeps and buzzes of life-saving machines.

Sometimes it was only my alarm clock that brought those

sessions to an abrupt end. It was supposed to wake me up at two fifteen for my shift at *Good Morning Britain*. But I hadn't slept, so had no alternative but to shake myself down, jump into the shower, as if it were a portal between the two worlds, and head into work. Jumping backwards and forwards between my two worlds was dizzying, exhausting and heartbreaking.

I tried to focus on my daily working life on TV and radio. On air at *Good Morning Britain*, I was doing what I hoped I had done for the last twenty years: trying to hold politicians and authority to account, and help others to tell their stories in their own way. And that felt good.

I knew that my situation – trying to carry on despite the devastation Covid had brought to our family – wasn't unique. Hundreds of thousands were doing the same. It helped me to think that if my voice on TV could speak for them, it might give them some relief too, reinforcing the idea that we are not alone. On Smooth it was wonderful to feel I was helping people to escape the misery with music – radio is such a great way to connect! The listeners knew what I was going through and reacted with so much support. I was deeply moved. I knew what they were going through, separated from their loved ones, millions of little islands trying to keep going. If I could bring joy, a smile or a memory from playing a favourite song or by sharing a joke or observation about the weird, frightening world in which we were living, then that might help – and helping felt good.

Likewise, with Derek and his world of doctors I tried to find a similar degree of purpose. I had always felt helpless, trusting in the energy, experience and knowledge of the doctors to bring him back to us. But now, knowing they too were navigating the unknown, as the new long-term effects of Covid began to reveal themselves across the world, I felt almost more included. And I was an expert in something they weren't: I was an expert in Derek.

With each FaceTime call I was still looking for something that only I would know: a flicker, a twitch, a glance. After all, they only knew a post-Covid Derek in his passive semi-conscious state. I knew it all. If I spotted anything, no matter how small, I always let the team know. Of course it was often impossible for them to judge whether it was involuntary or he was trying to communicate. But they always noted it down. At last, I felt I was contributing to the mapping of his progress.

Sometimes I couldn't control my emotions or keep my focus. My fear for Derek and for all our futures was enormous, and the only way I could control these overwhelming moments was by 'staying in lane'. It became my new mantra. If someone at work, or out and about, asked how Derek or I was doing, I would say, with a laugh, 'Don't ask! We'll be here all day and we'll never get on air!' I knew if I started talking about what was happening in the clinical world, all the fear, all the uncertainty would surge up and stop me functioning. I had to stay focused on the world I was in at that time. I said it so often that it started to catch on with people around me. My boss at Smooth Radio suddenly found that when anyone went off on a tangent during a business Zoom, she would start shouting, 'Stay in lane! We have to stay in lane!'

Summer started to bleed into autumn, and as the days got shorter it became harder and harder to focus, to keep hope alive. The light at the end of the tunnel was there, but the tunnel seemed to get longer. I could feel in my bones that somewhere deep inside me the enemy of hope – *despair* – was bubbling up. And worse than that, I could sense it was happening to people all around me too.

We had gone into the first lockdown as a nation thinking it was short-term, dramatic, almost interesting as a communal experience and we came out of it sincerely believing that life would get back to some kind of normal before too long. Shops were opening, pubs and restaurants doing a roaring trade, and, to everyone's relief, hairdressers were back in business. Schools allowed youngsters to mix, giving parents a break from home schooling. Hope was busting out all over! Could it be that we *would* actually get through this? Was there an end in sight? Hey, could this *really* be over by Christmas?

With alarming speed the new confidence started to slip away. The infection rates went up, as did the number of hospitalizations. Schools had to send home swathes of students to self-isolate, causing chaos for working parents, and university students found themselves effectively still home learning but far from home, and from their support networks.

Every day new rules and restrictions were introduced as the authorities struggled to get the infection rates under control, trying to balance safety with keeping the economy going. Those in industries like hospitality, who had previously been seen as champions driving the economy forward, suddenly found themselves accused of running pockets of infection, despite spending thousands to meet the new rules.

Resentment crept in. The Dominic Cummings debacle had already shattered the idea that we were all in the same boat, damaging trust irreparably. People asked themselves why they should stick to the rules if the politicians who made them were flouting them. Neighbours started to resent neighbours, wondering why some could work when they couldn't, why some occupations were suddenly seen as less important at best or dangerous at worst. When the chancellor, Rishi Sunak, talked about 'viable jobs' being supported, he infuriated those who found themselves, through no fault of their own, in apparently 'unviable' roles.

We were encouraged to confront people we knew were breaking the rules, and maybe it was the right thing to do to tackle the pandemic but it did nothing for the mood of togetherness and community that had been such a positive force through the first lockdown. There was a sense of trouble brewing, while commentators talked about the need to 'get a hold of things' and of the fear of riots on the streets if even more restrictions were imposed or if numbers went up. Suddenly it felt as if the world was unravelling. People's frustrations were bubbling up into anger: at the authorities, at each other, at the world.

It was frightening – and anger often is frightening because it's an emotion that shows a lack of self-control. We fear where anger may lead. A burst of anger at a stranger who has knocked your pint might feel good in the moment, but it can have disastrous consequences, especially for those caught in the crossfire.

This is something Derek and I talked a lot about. His psychotherapy sessions provided a safe and appropriate place for his clients to be angry without being judged. It was part of his job to help them release that anger, to get it out without harming others, and *then* to help them analyse what was driving it.

'Is it really true that you're this unhappy because your partner goes to the gym every Friday or is it because you feel neglected? Is it that particular new outfit which represents everything wrong with your marriage, or is it really that you think they don't realize how much effort you've made to earn the household money? Are you struggling to sustain that effort and feeling ashamed you can't do more? Could it be that getting angry with your partner is a way of avoiding those feelings within yourself?'

These were the sorts of questions that Derek had been trained to ask about anger, so he found it relatively easy to look deeper, to see what else might be there. Since childhood I had very rarely seen anger at all so it often terrified me.

I didn't grow up in an angry house. In fact, I can't remember my parents ever having a row in front of my brother and me. The closest we ever came to it was one year as we drove to Wales for our annual family camping holiday. There was no satnav back then, and my mum was navigating, Ordnance Survey map balanced precariously on her lap. She missed calling out the turning off the motorway and my dad snapped, 'Oh, Mary, for God's sake,' out of frustrated tension. To our horror she snapped back, 'OK OK! I'm doing my best.'

It was nothing really, something other families see every few hours. But the tone was so angry, different from what we were used to, that my brother Matthew and I looked at each other in the back seat, disturbed by this rip in the fabric of our normality. The fact that we still remember it to this day says it all.

Living with parents who got on so well was a peaceful and loving way to grow up and I'm very grateful for it. But I suppose if there was one downside it was that I hadn't learnt to put anger into context. I would be at a friend's house hearing their parents going hammer and tongs, shouting at each other, and ask, 'Are you OK? That sounds scary.'

'Oh, they're always bickering like that,' my friend would say. 'They'll be laughing in a minute.' And indeed they were.

When I first met Derek, he had very strong views on anger and expressed them – well – angrily. 'Anger is *good* for you,' he told me. 'It gets frustration out of the system.' After a big old rant about something (often my untidiness!) you could see him physically relax. 'That's better,' he would say.

'It's all right for you,' I would reply, 'but after that performance I'm all in a whirl!'

'Kate, just because I'm angry it doesn't mean I don't love you any more. It doesn't mean anything more than I'm cross about this one particular thing. It's much better to get it out, or otherwise it will turn into bitterness, resentment, despair ... which are all so much unhealthier. It's just an emotion.

You have to free it so that you can own it. Then you can control it.'

In time I came to see that he was right. He would use the anger to fire himself up to take on new challenges and free himself from more negative emotions.

My friend Clare had given me a self-help book to read, and I found myself flicking through it in bed one night, when my eye landed on a table of emotions. At the bottom were depression, apathy, despair. Then it worked up the scale, passing through hope to optimism to confidence to joy. It struck a chord. The book explained that when you look at the range of human emotions, you shouldn't see one as better than another, or beat yourself up about which one you're feeling: you just notice how you feel and what each emotion gives you. Anger, it explained, can be such a rewarding emotion to those who feel helpless and desperate, because if you're feeling angry, it's a powerful emotion that you're directing outwards; helplessness and despair tend to be directed inwards.

As I struggled to stay positive, I thought a lot about not giving in to despair at the lack of change, at the uncertainty of whether Derek could ever make it back to us. Maybe I could do with releasing a bit of anger, I thought. But for anger to be truly liberating, to get that healing rush, you have to have something to be angry about. You have to have something to blame, to focus on.

You often see parents doing this with their children, particularly toddlers. A small child will fall over and bump their head or graze their knee. The child is crying in pain, but also in shock, and wants Mum or Dad to make it better. Arguably, the pain in that instant is felt far more intensely by the parent than the child: nothing cuts as deeply as hearing your child cry, and when a cuddle doesn't stop the tears, the pain becomes impossible to bear. It's then you often see something strange, or it has always seemed strange to me: the parent blames the pavement, the table or whatever it is that the child has hurt itself on. The adult will so often say, 'Oh no, naughty pavement. Naughty pavement doing that to your knee. Let's tell that pavement off. We're cross with it. Let's give it a smack. Naughty pavement, don't ever do that again.'

I can remember being in a park once with Derek (pre-Darcey and Billy) when a dad was doing just that with his little boy.

'Why do people do that?' I asked Derek. 'Why do they have to turn something that's just an accident into something else's fault? Why does there have to be blame? Things go wrong in life. Isn't it better to teach your children you just have to suck it up and get on with it? Isn't it teaching kids not to accept that bad stuff happens? What's worse, they're teaching them to feel better by *hitting*?'

'Oh God,' he laughed, 'you're such a *Garraway*.' He and the children say it to me all the time, and it usually means I'm being *too* nice, wanting the world to be cosy, happy, Disney perfect.

'I do love this quality about you, you know, but just because you don't seem to relish ever getting angry, it doesn't mean that the rest of us don't. Anger feels good sometimes. Yes, of course it's ridiculous to blame a pavement and of course we should all take personal responsibility, but if it's easier to blame a pavement, if it gets you through the moment, why not? As long as you don't get consumed by anger and blame – that's when the danger sets in …'

By not getting angry, by trying to stay calm and collected, was I in danger of wrapping myself in despair? And would it come out in a more dangerous way, for me and for Darcey and Billy too?

I could see that despair was creeping up on them. They missed their dad so much and the emotionless, passive, staring person they saw on FaceTime was no comfort. At first it had really helped to do the video calls. They had never been allowed to visit the hospital, so their imaginations had been running riot, and it had helped to see him on the screen. I was surprised by how they managed, in the amazing way that kids do, to look past the tubes and the weight loss, seeing only their dad: they loved him and he was alive. They were brilliant at just chatting away to the nothingness. It was genuinely impressive and I was so proud of them.

But it was harder and harder for them when they were getting nothing back. Darcey loved debating with Derek – they would row for hours about everything from capital punishment to whether teenagers should run for office, the virtues of YouTube over reading books, and whether under-eighteens should be allowed to get tattoos. I'll leave you to guess who was arguing for what! They loved it. The debates would become more and more frenzied, their arguments for and against more extreme and ridiculous. Doors would be slammed, opened again and they'd be back for more, always ending in laughter if not agreement.

Now when Darcey tried to get her message through to Derek on FaceTime, she used her old tactics, trying to wind him up, trying to shock. She even started getting angry with him directly. 'Dad, enough is enough. I'm getting cross with you now. WAKE UP,' she once shouted so loudly into the iPad that I jumped out of my skin, looking at her in disbelief but also wondering if it had worked. I watched her, staring at the screen for what seemed like an age, waiting for a reaction. And when nothing came she sighed, told him she loved him and would chat tomorrow.

'Worth a try,' she said to me, after she signed off. I knew she was disappointed but determined not to show it to me or him.

I tried to fill the gap and start debates with Darcey, rising to the challenge of her shock tactics. But she just rolled her eyes. 'Give it up, Mum. No one believes you're really angry. You don't even have an angry voice. You're just too *reasonable* – it's no fun.' Who knew being reasonable was such a crime? Sometimes as a parent you just can't win.

I remembered having similar feelings about 'reasonable' conversations with my mum and dad. I would come home from school with a playground drama. 'Jenny said my shoes were ugly and made me look stupid' or some such. I was hurt, embarrassed and full of self-doubt. *Were* my shoes ugly? *Did* I look stupid?

At this point some parents would have flown into a hurt rage. 'How *dare* that child make my daughter cry?' They would have said that Jenny was a horrible little girl, that, no, my shoes weren't ugly, in fact Jenny's were far uglier and she was just jealous. 'I'm having a word with her parents. She can't get away with this!' or versions of that would have been wielded. I'm sure that in most cases that would have been distinctly unhelpful and probably led to far worse pain than the initial comment.

My parents would explain that Jenny had only said it because she was miserable, that her mum and dad were getting divorced, that life at home was difficult, that she was unsettled, unhappy or whatever, and it was coming out as meanness to me. Sometimes when you're miserable, almost without knowing it you want others to be miserable too, my parents would explain. And I got it. And, of course, without realizing it, I then felt bad for Jenny. I couldn't blame her for being mean, because now I understood where it had come from.

I turned the anger inwards: I felt guilty because my life was nicer than hers, that my mum and dad loved each other, that my home was stable. I was too grateful. I couldn't let the anger out. Anger was averted, but was *all* negative emotion?

I don't *blame* my parents, by the way. They were teaching me valuable lessons that have helped me through so much in life. It's probably one of the reasons I do what I do as a journalist and interviewer: their way of thinking, putting yourself in other people's shoes, has always helped me to empathize, to see the other side of the argument. But as I've grown older, I've been able to see that giving anger its moment is important too. And right now Darcey needed hers.

Darcey didn't want reason. She didn't want to be told she was lucky that her dad was still alive when others had died. It was the situation *her* dad was in that was making her angry, and she wanted licence to scream at the top of her voice, fury spilling from her that he had fallen sick at all.

And she wasn't alone: across the nation it felt as if no one wanted 'reasonable' when life was just too infuriating. Life had become too unreasonable to be reasonable about. The rumours of the second wave seemed to be becoming reality, which seemed cripplingly unfair when so many had sacrificed so much to avoid it. You could see the frustration and rage bubbling up on the streets as some would panic about not being given enough space to walk two metres apart, while others resisted the requests to wear masks. We saw it on the headlines as lockdown measures changed at the drop of a hat, requiring huge shifts and sacrifices on what appeared to some like unexplained governmental whims. When I interviewed politicians, the reaction from viewers was angry too. During the first wave there was a craving to hear what they had to say: so many tuned into those daily government press conferences, hanging on every word, the sense of a wartime briefing about the whole thing. We all understood the circumstances were exceptional, the stakes incredibly high, the situation we were facing unknown.

We were running out of patience, and the lack of clarity had started to look like incompetence. From the frequency with which tier systems, quarantine rules and local furlough schemes chopped and changed, the system wasn't running seamlessly, and 'We're doing all we can' started to sound like an excuse, not an explanation. I could feel the viewers' blood boiling when systems like the Serco Test and Trace were clearly not 'world class', as we had been promised. But no one would admit it, and the government kept hiding from these blatant truths. 'Who are you trying to kid? Do you think we're idiots?' you could hear people screaming at the TV. The trust was gone.

The national anger continued to bubble as we headed towards Christmas with rules changing and new laws seemingly being brought in all of the time. Increasingly, I felt surrounded by rage. The frustration many felt was affecting our collective mental health. People wanted to get on with their lives. They had lost jobs, businesses, careers they had worked their lives for, in respect of an illness about which some were now asking, 'Is it any worse than flu?'

Now, horror of horrors, it looked like Christmas, the spot on the horizon that promised a release from the drudgery and misery, was going to be cancelled. And, even worse, there was unlikely to be a full stop to the pain at the end of the year. We had taken comfort in saying, 'Let's just get this hideous year out of the way, say goodbye to 2020, and move on.'

We were realizing that 2021 wasn't going to be a fresh dawn but an extension to the long black night. The new lockdown left few avenues to turn the rage into something concrete, something positive for the future. We were left with this aching emptiness, despair, and nowhere to put it.

The situation in Manchester when the local lockdowns and highest tier allocations were announced was a good example of anger being put to a use that had a tangible result. Opposition parties had broadly stood by the government at the beginning: it was a national emergency. Now the gloves were off. Labour local mayor Andy Burnham was refusing to speak with the usual platitudes – not even making much pretence at politeness! – but instead appearing on news broadcast after news broadcast visibly seething with rage. Whether his stand-off delivered a better result for the people of Manchester than quiet negotiations the political experts will debate for ever, but there is no doubt it made the people there *feel* better. To see someone fighting their cause, unleashing righteous anger and focusing it on the government was a sweet release.

I began to understand that I needed a bit of the sweet release of rage. After all, it wasn't that I didn't *feel* anger. Of *course* I had anger inside, even though I might not be showing it. Anger that Derek had got sick in the first place, anger that because he was in the first wave he had missed out on treatments that might have saved him from the worst of the Covid damage, anger that he'd missed out on trials. But alongside those flashes of anger there was guilt because I knew he might have died and I had so very much to be grateful for. Also, it was no one's *fault*. There was no one to blame. The doctors were fighting a war against an unknown enemy and had saved his life. How could I feel anything other than incredibly lucky? Anger seemed criminally ungrateful.

'You *should* be angry,' said my friend Chris Hawkins, from BBC Radio 6 Music. 'I'm furious for you, so you have every right to be angry for yourself. Frankly, if I could get my hands on that virus I'd knock seven bells out of it.'

Chris is the most peace-loving, considerate and gentle man, and the idea of him punching the virus with all his might, fists flying and face red with fury, was so incongruous it made me giggle.

'Ye-es – the only trouble is how do you punch a microscopic virus particle that you can't see?' I wondered. And we both laughed.

'I guess that's what we're all working out, doctors, politicians, all of us. How to punch Covid out,' said Chris. 'But if anyone could knock Covid out cold, it's Darcey. Remember what she's like with piñatas at kids' parties? She takes no prisoners.'

He was right and, better still, he gave me an idea. I went online and, sure enough, it was possible to buy a piñata shaped like a giant version of the coronavirus! I ordered one immediately. It arrived within a couple of days and we filled it with chocolates and just let loose. It was hilarious: shrieks across the garden, kids charging at the piñata, chocolates flying everywhere. Very satisfying indeed.

Once again I was reminded that anger is a great way to alleviate panic, fear or despair when you feel their icy grip on you. The trick, I now understood, is to allow yourself to feel anger when you do, and to acknowledge it, to think, This anger is helping me to cope. I can see why it's here. But also to grasp why it's not that helpful in the long term and let it go. Because if you stay in anger, it will pull you down, possibly indefinitely.

History has shown us that anger can be a huge driving force for good *and* bad. It can be an incredible motivator to create change that doesn't just relieve your own despair but lifts others out of it too. But if you let it consume you, it can take you down a very dangerous track. I remember my history professor at college, who was Jewish, explaining the successful rise of the Nazi Party between the two world wars was due to the collective desire of a country to relieve itself of the miserable situation it was in, to relieve the shame the world had placed on it after it had lost the First World War, and to find someone other than itself to blame. It might sound 'out there' or too simplistic, but his argument got us thinking. A hundred years ago, Germany was on its knees economically. The country had lost a war, lost any pride, was consumed with a kind of national shame and despair. Then the Nazi Party popped up, with all its glamour, its huge, confident, colourful rallies, and its promise of making Germany great again, just what the incumbent government wasn't delivering.

And when the Nazi Party presented rage at the Jews, it gave the population someone to blame for their misery. The professor argued that this had led the nation and ultimately the world down a very dark path. Over the years, political parties have often used this as a tactic: blame as a fire for collective action. Here, parties like the National Front have done similar, blaming economic worry on immigration: 'Can't get a job? Blame those immigrants. It's their fault. They've taken yours.'

I was trying to acknowledge my anger and let it lift me

out of the despair I felt that Derek couldn't make it back to us, without letting it consume me and, of course, without blaming anyone. Anger can be so useful: a driver, and a relief from the helplessness of feeling eternally sad. I was trying to use it to fuel me to throw myself into the practical: another phone call, another visit, another day at work. It pushed me through.

And I realized, as the days passed, I had seen other families do this as a response to immense grief and pain. Over the years I have interviewed many families of children who have been killed, and seen anger manifesting in a variety of ways. Some have turned to making a change in the law, and others have invested all of that fuel in charity work. But others have let it destroy them, unable to break out of the bitter hold it has on them. If you sit with your anger for too long, it can eat you up, turn into bitterness, hold you back in a mire of pain. The parents who survived the worst of these awful circumstances had so often got hold of this fact, trying to turn anger into something positive.

Now, I had to use it to fire me to keep me going, to help alleviate the helplessness, to lift me out of despair. I had to keep believing that Derek could make it back, that he could express, that he could feel. That I would see the fire, the anger in his eyes again. Seeing that anger would be pure joy.

Chapter 11

Determination and Delusion

If it was determination that was needed, I knew I had buckets of that. Well, I like to think of it as determination. I suspect my friends would say I'm just plain stubborn. Anyway, I always flatly refuse to give up on anything I've started. I prefer to think of it as stamina – so much more attractive than stubbornness!

I never shone at sports at school, I was never first to be picked for a team, but I always did OK at cross-country running. Why? Because I kept going. I even managed to come second in an inter-school competition as a teenager. The weather was so bad that day but, of course, the contest wasn't cancelled, thanks to the classic British 'Get out there – it'll do you good!' attitude. So, as the rain pelted down, the faster runners than me wading through the thick mud just thought, Stuff this for a game of soldiers, and pulled out, but I ploughed on. One foot in front of the other. Until I came second.

As I clutched my silver medal proudly on the school bus home, my PE teacher had a bemused expression, clearly trying to figure out what had led to my mini triumph. After a while, she suddenly perked up.

'You, Kathryn [as I was called back then] are a classic case of the tortoise and the hare. You just keep plodding on. It's not flashy, it's not pretty but it *does* get you there.'

Clearly she was comparing me with the tortoise – not the ideal description of yourself for a teenager – and I must have looked downcast.

'It's a compliment!' she added. 'It means you'll win through in the end. The great thing about you is that you don't mind looking like an idiot – and you're tougher than you look. The others all struggled, hated being cold and wet, but you seemed to thrive on it.'

It wasn't the kind of rewarding speech I'd been looking for from the coach, but even then I understood what she meant. It wasn't that I loved hardship – I always run towards cosy comfort – but when there doesn't seem much choice, you just have to get on with it, don't you? A bit of cold and rain *doesn't* kill you, so crack on. That was the way I'd been brought up, and never thought to question it.

There's no doubt that this attitude went on to help me in my working life. It meant I was prepared to stand in the cold longer than anyone else to get a story, to make that extra phone call, to get in that bit earlier for a shift, to skip an extra hour's sleep or a fun night out with friends. It's a no-pain-no-gain work ethic that might not work for every-one, but it seems to have worked for me. Others perhaps had more talent to get them there without the pain, but I always knew I'd have to work harder and longer to achieve the same result. I was indeed the tortoise.

There have been times in my personal life when this attitude hasn't helped. For instance, in my relationships: I would often stick at them long after others would have got out, hanging in there, trying to fix things, believing if I could just try harder, look better, it could still all work out beautifully. Friends would tell me to give up, but I'd always think, Nothing's ever perfect, you have to work at it. How much of it is my fault? What if I just did this? Or that? Then he's sure to see that we're actually meant to be!

It must have been bewildering for the guys involved – I was almost suffocating them with love until eventually they ran for the hills. I, of course, was left broken-hearted, wondering what more I could possibly have done.

Now, as autumn crept on, I started to hear a tone in my friends' voices that reminded me of those old days: a shift from admiration at my determination to a gentle questioning as to whether I was clinging to a false reality. This time was it the delusion that Derek could come home? I could tell that the hope my friends had helped me to build up, that had kept me going this far, was now turning into concern that I was refusing to let go of a fantasy.

I even started to wonder myself – not that I ever for a second weakened in my determination to do everything I could to keep going for Derek and the kids. But I did think about the point at which I should start to let go, begin a kind of grieving for the person he had been rather than believing in the miracle of his return exactly as he was when he went into the hospital. My manifesting told me I had to believe as hard as I could in the best possible outcome, but at what point did reality come in?

There were days when the progress felt real but it was always a frustrating case of one step forward two steps back, then two steps forward one step back. And with no precedent of anyone else having recovered from this scale of Covid damage, it was impossible to be confident that there *was* an upward trajectory. It was such a mountain to climb for Derek to get back to us, and without knowing if reaching the summit was possible, the endeavour felt doubly hard. For every bit of progress, there was a reason why it wasn't progress: it could just be involuntary, it could be a twitch, it could be survival instinct, it could be a learnt reaction rather than a real sign of the old Derek coming back.

I felt as if I was walking a tightrope between determination, hope and delusion. So much of the time I felt as if my belief was the only lifeline Derek had.

The incredible team working on him were the real lifeline, of course, but it was their responsibility to be factual, to stay scientific. There was no room for fantasy, for expectation, for hope: they had to grade everything, noting it without emotion, creating a scientific picture to rebuild him.

When we think of rehab, we tend to imagine someone who has to find their way back from a terrible car crash or a similar physical incident. We think of learning to walk or talk again, a mechanical process. But Derek's situation was a 'prolonged disorder of consciousness', so it was the mechanics but also the mind that we were trying to recover. He hadn't moved a muscle for months, so the team didn't know if he was paralysed by the effects of Covid or simply too weak to move after months of lying immobile. Part of the rehabilitation process was moving him to help improve the strength and flexibility of his body.

But immobilization also affects the brain. When we move our limbs, or take any physical action, our brain has to have the thought to do it – even if it's a lightning-fast response that we barely remember. But how and where we move our limbs also takes messages back to the brain. Is that pan hot? Is that ground stable? And so on. Messages are going back and forth all the time.

The rehabilitation team were moving Derek in the hope of stimulating these messages to go both ways. Perhaps moving him would trigger the brain to make more movements. So they moved him, every day, very gently back and forth. This worked his muscles so that he was rebuilding strength, and served the invaluable neurological purpose of reminding his brain of what it had to do, hoping to trigger it into the ability to move.

He had been lying flat for so long that his muscles were at risk of seizing up entirely, which was what happened to patients years ago. Someone would fall into a coma, through accident or disease, and would be left lying still. Doctors didn't understand back then that the patient *needed* to move to know *how* to move. Muscles and ligaments would freeze.

There was a limited period before that happened to Derek so the team had to try every trick in the book. At one point they used Botox to relax his muscles, which allowed them to move him more easily. The children and I chuckled about this. Derek was appalled by Botox for cosmetic improvement as he thought it made people look weird – and now he was getting it, if for different reasons.

As well as movement and Botox, the team also used gravity. After lying flat for so long Derek had not felt gravity when he was upright; bearing weight is vital to strengthening muscles and potentially triggering awakening. The brain knows when the body is upright so would this help to bring him back?

The hospital has a piece of kit called a tilt table, a flat bed to which Derek was strapped. Through the use of hydraulics, it would gradually start tilting him into a more vertical position so that he could begin to feel gravity run down from his head through his body, in his muscles, sinews, blood vessels. Even this change in position would have a huge effect on how his heart was working. The aim was to turn him to near ninety degrees so that he was effectively standing, so he could feel the pull of gravity without needing to support himself. And the hospital would monitor every vital organ as they did this.

At first, even when he was moved by just twelve degrees, his blood pressure dropped drastically – he effectively passed out – and he had to be returned to the horizontal. His vascular system was no longer strong enough to keep the blood flowing. They had to adjust his medication, to control his blood pressure, and gradually keep going. After a while, they could get him to sixty degrees, and this was considered great progress – someone semi-conscious like Derek wouldn't be able to get fully upright: they would feel as though they were falling forward. Once they managed to get him almost vertical they could then begin to use different therapies.

They had a contraption that could wrap around Derek's limbs and mechanically move his arms and legs in a rotating rhythm to simulate and stimulate a walking action. It made him look like a robot. It was frightening to watch him, via FaceTime, being moved by a machine, his stick-thin legs clearly unable to bear weight, his expressionless staring eyes, as if he wasn't there, as if he'd been taken over by artificial intelligence, his body snatched. Even though he wasn't fully conscious, I thought he must have been aware of the movement and it must have been terrifying for him to be so vulnerable, so out of control in his own body. All the time he was being moved in these machines, the teams were talking to him, explaining what was happening, and why they were doing it. They wanted him to connect with their instruction, to help him be more present in his own body.

After one of these sessions, which I had found so disturbing, I talked to one of my doctor friends outside the team and explained what had happened.

'Kate, it's a miracle he's survived … but maybe he's one of those who wasn't meant to survive.'

What was he saying? That it would have been better if Derek had died?

'No way,' I said. 'I'm not accepting that. While there's life there's hope, and even the doctors say they don't know. It's all too unknown. There's still a chance that Derek *can* be the exception. I'm not going to give up. I'm *determined*.'

But it had been clear that he was wondering if I was deluded and needed to start accepting the truth.

Was I wrong to keep going? *Was* it doing Derek any favours, my persistence? In the past I have interviewed parents who have been told by doctors that their gravely ill child is definitely not going to recover. In these cases parents are often convinced there is hope, sometimes taking legal action to keep life support going, while doctors argue that it's wrong to keep a child alive when they may be in pain. Was *this* what I was facing? Was I doing *this* to Derek? Was I being selfish, trying to hang on to him for my sake, for the sake of the children, for the people who loved him? Was I actually keeping him trapped in a prison? Some days I was haunted by the idea that he might be locked in, in pain, with no chance of showing it.

But even if the team caring for Derek were constantly cautious about raising my expectations, stopping me having false hope, they didn't hold back in doing everything they could to help his recovery. Some of the things they thought of blew my mind, only serving to give me more hope, regardless of how they were trying to contain it in me. Over the weeks and months their precise, compassionate care helped to manage infections while allowing small parts of him to recover over time. Gradually they got him off kidney dialysis, and then carefully – with the usual two steps forward, one step back – they decreased the amount of support he was getting from the ventilator, until they could risk letting him breathe alone. At this point, he was in a state of minimum consciousness, still technically in a coma but not as we think of it, which for most people is probably completely unconscious. As a result, the team had to see which of his involuntary life-saving processes could work without machines.

Before they could remove the tracheotomy tube in his throat, they had to check his swallow action: if he couldn't swallow independently, he would choke on his saliva. To check this, they put a tiny amount of ice cream in his mouth. The cold of the ice cream would feel so different from saliva, but would he notice? If he sensed a difference, a reflex action to swallow should kick in. We all waited with bated breath as they repeated the test, day after day. At first, he didn't notice a thing – and then one day he did. And after a couple of weeks he seemed to gobble it down! Was it hunger, his body's instinct to feed itself after so many weeks of being fed by tubes? Or was Derek simply enjoying a taste of ice cream after such a joyless few months? We couldn't know, until he could express himself better.

The team reassured me that his brain signals weren't showing signs of distress, that his heart rate was under control and that he didn't seem to be feeling any pain, but until he established some form of communication I couldn't be sure. A separate team was trying to build communication, which would be the first step in trying to haul his mind back now that his body was gaining strength and independence. They were trying different ways to see if he might be able to respond. Blink once for yes, twice for no. Look left for yes, right for no. Squeeze my hand, move your thumb. Anything.

Sometimes he seemed to react but then days would pass, weeks even, when he didn't. Had previous results been a fluke? Had they meant anything at all?

I was asked to bring in more pictures of the family to see if they would trigger anything. I had to write on the back of each image who the people pictured were so that staff could chat to him about it. There were also familiar things around him that were tactile to trigger touch and brain connection. He had a few ceramic stones he had bought in San Francisco when studying there. They were painted with bright colours, images of rainbows, storm clouds and the like on the front, with words written on the back. The idea is that whichever picture you're drawn to, when you turn the stone to reveal the word, it will tell you the mood you're in. It was a hippie, fortune-teller gimmick, but they were also very satisfying to touch. The children had loved playing with them when they were small, and a few had got broken so Derek had taken them to his office in town and would run his fingers through them as he concentrated on an idea or a gnarly phone call. I suppose they served the same purpose for him as worry beads. I thought they might trigger memories as well as sensory stimulation, and the occupational therapists used them in sessions.

They positioned the stones under his right hand so he was touching them and somehow managed to get his head at an angle so he could also see them. Again, the occupational therapist was talking to him all the time, reading out from the notes I had given them about where he'd got the stones, the stories behind them, trying to stimulate memory.

I had already told them that his eyesight had been poor even before he had contracted Covid. He needed glasses to see anything clearly. It was one of his stupid jokes that when he woke up he would turn to me in bed and say, 'My God, you look beautiful,' then put his glasses on and recoil, shrieking, 'Jeez!'

The doctors already knew that Covid could affect sight, and some patients had been left blind or partially sighted, so we had no idea what Derek could see now – but it was certainly logical that Covid hadn't improved his sight. Putting his glasses on must help a little bit. One day he was staring at the stones with his glasses in place and the occupational therapist observed that his eyes were wide open, staring as if trying to draw in every bit of what he saw, up and into his brain. He didn't appear to be reacting to anything she was saying, just staring … staring … moving thumb and forefinger over the ceramic stones. She carried on chatting away, keeping the narrative going, trying to build communication and connection.

The team who work with patients in prolonged disorders of consciousness are the most extraordinary people. All of them – doctors, nurses, therapists, carers, porters – play their part, with a relentless projection of positivity. Their ability to be cheerful, to chat in a lively manner at a virtual vacuum, to keep treating someone in that state with such dignity and humanity, is amazing. For most people, talking to someone who doesn't respond would be like talking to nothing: we would start to drift away, go into our own thoughts, but they keep going, projecting out, knowing it's the key to bringing someone back.

And as this occupational therapist was chatting away, she noticed that because of the strange angle that Derek was propped up at, his glasses had started to slide down his nose and were precariously perched on its very end.

'Ooh, Derek,' she said, 'what's happened to your glasses? They're making a bid for freedom! That won't do, will it? Let's push those glasses back on your nose.'

And as she said this, she began to stand up, about to move towards him to push up his glasses. But before she got anywhere near him, something extraordinary happened: Derek reached up with his right hand and pushed them back himself. She stopped in her tracks, almost wondering if her eyes had deceived her. She tried to get him to do it again, moving his glasses back down. Nothing. She couldn't get him to repeat it for days, weeks afterwards. But it had happened.

She rang me excitedly to explain. 'Oh my! So he knows he's wearing glasses and knows how to put them back up – that movement, that coordination, it's unbelievable!'

'That means he's there! That he understands he's him ...' I said, tears welling in my eyes with relief.

'Well, yes and no,' she said. 'It shows he can do it, but only instinctively. The pathway in his brain that knows how to put glasses back up is there, but he's been doing that for decades. Glasses slip down, he slides them back up, it's hardwired in, but he can't do it consciously. That's what we need to work on.'

Meanwhile, we had our own 'rehab team' going on FaceTime. I would talk to Derek constantly, sometimes just relaying my day, even though I was doing very little. I would give him updates on the family, the kids, anything that would seem familiar. Something to normalize the situation, to give him a sense of who he was beyond someone just stuck in that alien world. Other times, I would test him to see if I could get any reaction: nothing. He was frozen.

Then one day I spotted something. Derek has an expression he wore when he was concentrating, writing at his computer, a working expression. He never had it when he was watching a movie or relaxing reading a book, only when he was trying to draw something out of his mind. It was similar to a child in school concentrating at their desk: sometimes they stick their tongue out of the side of their mouth, not realizing they're doing it. Derek would curl his top lip up, almost as if he were pursing his lips and rubbing them on his nose. It was weird – and deeply unattractive! And it drove me mad initially but then it became a cute quirk that was very much him.

On one of those FaceTimes, I was chatting to him, encouraging him, telling him I knew he was in there. He was staring hard at the screen, his eyes wide, maybe, I sensed, trying to focus too. Then suddenly he curled his lip and made his focusing expression, his eyes fixed on me. It was like a miracle! The first flash of the old Derek.

'Thank you! Thank you! I can see you're in there! I always knew it,' I cried, into the iPad.

I called the nurses into the room to see it too. But it was gone. Maybe their movement had broken his concentration. Maybe he was just too tired to continue and had slipped back down, deeper into unconsciousness. But I had seen it. There was no mistaking it in my mind.

I told the neurologist in charge. I could immediately tell he wasn't as excited as I was, pausing for a long time after I described the moment to him.

'I think we have to be careful we don't get carried away here, Kate,' he said. 'If you think about it, this is an involuntary action. He might have done it all his life. He might just be concentrating because there is a light flickering in front of him, because you are a voice that is talking to him all the time, because you're without a mask as you're using FaceTime and not in the room. That alone is different from the people caring for him. He might be trying to work things out, like a baby curious at a sparkly light. It doesn't mean he knows you, or knows what it is. He might not know the significance. It doesn't mean he's attached to you in any other way than that you're there in front of him.'

A pause, while I tried to absorb this blanket of caution.

'But it's definitely something to note. All of these things really help us, Kate, because it helps us gauge a reaction to what we're doing. It helps us to form a picture.'

In the face of these dampened expectations, I felt the need to widen the circle of people talking to him. If there were more people to assess, more people who knew him, then surely there would be different ways to spot the signs of his emergence. His mum wasn't keen as she felt Derek wouldn't want his friends to see him so vulnerable. I knew she was thinking of the Derek who had been there before – proud, always wanting to put on a show of bravado, not wanting people to think he was on his uppers. And he couldn't possibly have been more on his uppers than he was at the moment. I understood her protectiveness so suggested she try talking to him herself.

She agreed, so I persuaded the team at the hospital to allow his mum and dad to speak to him. He might need someone other than me and the kids – after all, he might not even remember us. I might be as much of a stranger talking to him as the therapists in masks who were in and out all day. Your mother's voice is the first you hear when you're born, a voice whose rhythm and tone you've been familiar with while still in the womb. She is the first person you connect with, and on such a primal level. If anyone could trigger recognition, surely it would be her.

But she was nervous, terrified, at what she would see. She had coped so well up to now, getting used to talking to him on the phone while it was held to his ear, but this was often not possible as the hospital was so busy. Seeing Derek would make his situation, the devastation that had taken place, very real. I knew all about that from my first visit, so I asked the team to keep the iPad camera on Derek's face. Then there was the practical problem of teaching his mum how to use an iPad. She'd be the first to admit she's no technical whizz kid. She can't text on a mobile and has never used a computer. Di, Derek's sister, lent her one, and sat outside on the front porch, teaching her the basics.

On one of these lessons they called me, hooting with laughter at how Chrina had finally been dragged into the twenty-first century, and I could tell with relief that they were happy to be doing something to help, to be feeling a little less cut off. Derek's mum was too nervous to go first, so Di did it, reassuring her that it was OK, and the next night his other sister, Sue, called. Then his mum. They kept up that rota, alternating every three nights and continuing to this day. For the first few weeks Derek's mum would sob after coming off the call, heartbroken at seeing him in that state. But each time it got better, and she did heroic work at holding it together when she was talking to him. I was so proud of her and all that they were doing.

It helped to have others to share what I was noticing on these FaceTimes. We would spend ages reporting back to each other any little signs we might have seen. Sometimes they thought they had seen mannerisms they recognized, which renewed our determination to keep going.

I also started to record my FaceTimes as the emotion of talking to him and my desire to project positivity meant that I couldn't study his face properly at the same time. I would watch them again and again, looking for anything that might be useful or recognizable. I would ask him to move something that I knew he could, such as his thumb, then wait and see. Sometimes it seemed he did, but at others it didn't. Weeks went on like this: stop, start; hope, doubt; determination, and the fear of delusion.

The more optimistic members of the team at the hospital explained that this inconsistency could be exhaustion, which was positive. The rehab they were giving him, moving him around so often, might not have seemed much – but, they explained, to Derek ten minutes of it would have been the equivalent of three marathons back to back. Some days he was just too exhausted to respond to anything. They explained that this wasn't just physical, it was mental too. His brain was now trying to communicate, as well as trying to work his body again. Some days he just slept and slept. Similarly, they realized that after months of being in an induced coma with no idea of day or night, he had to relearn how to tell the difference between the two. Sometimes he slept all day only to be awake all night, then was clearly exhausted the next day.

The children were trying to make sense of it. One day Darcey asked, 'What happens if Dad never gets better? What if he just stays like this, silent and staring? What will it be like, him sitting in a corner of the room?'

It was heartbreaking that she was even having to wonder about this, let alone possibly have to face it.

'If he could just talk it would make all the difference,' she continued. 'I don't want him to be paralysed, but if he is I could cope, and I think he could too. As long as he can talk and laugh with us.'

'I just want him to have the same sense of humour, to know me,' said Billy.

I had nothing to reassure them, apart from a hug and to admit the truth.

'It's what I want too. We all do. But you know who wants it the most?'

They both looked at me, eyes wide. Who?

'Dad,' I said. 'Dad wants to come back to us more than anything, and he won't want to miss a thing.'

Darcey smiled. 'Yes! He'll be furious he's missed so much already!'

They were laughing now at the thought of his 'fury' at missing out on the summer of sunshine. I couldn't reassure them with certainty from the doctors, but I had the certainty of the love I knew their dad had for them.

The attempts to get him communicating continued. Some days it looked as if he could nod for 'yes'. But then he seemed to struggle with 'no'. As Billy said, he had had no trouble saying 'no' before so we assumed it wasn't for a lack of trying!

The team also did a series of tests on his vocal cords because the tubes had been down his throat for so long that they might have been damaged, which might prevent him from speaking. They needed to rule out physical damage before they worried about mental effort on his part. But the tests showed that, while there might have been a bit of damage, it could not have been the cause of the problem. Just because vocal cords can work physically, it doesn't mean someone can speak their thoughts: a signal from the brain has to shape the mouth and tongue to form a word; a signal from the brain has to direct the right word; and, of course, it has to *know* what you want to express.

Derek was not just learning how to shape words, but

learning language all over again, like a baby. But unlike a baby, with whom we assume there is no problem unless they fall behind their peers, we had no idea whether Derek could relearn language, or if he ever would. The team would try to get him to shape sounds, starting at the very beginning with ma-ma-ma and da-da-da. Often, he looked as if he was trying to copy what they had said … but no sound.

On FaceTime I occasionally thought he was trying to mouth words. His face had started to get some movement: he had gained some control over his tongue and lips from the ice cream and other therapies. But when I told the team at the hospital, they said he *might* be trying to mouth words or he might simply be watching my mouth and copying me. In addition, they pointed out that he might just be experiencing renewed sensation in his mouth, perhaps that strange sensation of feeling and no feeling, like pins and needles as your leg comes back to life after you've been sitting curled up on a chair.

Then, at last, came the breakthrough. One morning the physios were moving him, trying to stimulate feeling as they always did, and accompanying it with their usual friendly chit-chat. 'Let me know if this is uncomfortable,' and 'Let me know if anything hurts, Derek,' and so on. Out of the blue came a word. Clear and unmistakable.

'Pain.'

Not a mouthed word, not a whisper, but an actual sound, clear as a bell. 'Pain.'

Of course the team rang me immediately. Part of me was horrified that that could be his first word, that that must have been his prevalent thought or experience, if it was strong enough to prompt speech. Had he been feeling it all along but unable to express it? It seemed like torture to have been trapped in pain but unable to express it.

But it showed a brain connection, and this was incredible news. He had *felt something* and he *knew* and used the *right* word to articulate what it was. He had been able to send a signal to his mouth and throat to express it. Language! He had felt something, and he had told us! So simple, but so utterly profound.

He managed it again a few days later, when I was watching him have rehab on FaceTime. It wasn't very loud, but I could see the mouthing clearly, not once but twice. He had no expression, he showed no emotion, and he didn't look as if he was in any pain – he didn't wince or screw up his face – but there it was. The connection. A word used in context.

The neuropsychologist explained to me that it might be about finding the right motivation: if there was a sensation inside him that was strong enough, he could make the mental connection. And him saying, 'Pain,' seemed to have proved that. We just had to find the right motivation for more. The neuropsychologist explained that motivation didn't simply mean 'being bothered', as we might refer to the motivation to tidy the house or do the laundry. In this case it was a physical barrier called 'initiation' that the altered state of consciousness, the coma, had caused. Even if Derek wanted to, he couldn't get the signal out to make it happen, and this related to physical movement as well as communication. He warned me that this might mean that Derek had only basic survival instincts left: fight or flight; pain and avoiding it are vital for survival – that he might not be capable of higher thought.

I chose to see it as a breakthrough. Yes, just saying, 'Pain,' was a long way from the caring, sensitive, clever husband and father Derek had been before Covid, but it was a start. And I was convinced that this was what he would want me to think too. Up in his Thinking Room hung a sign, saying, 'No beginning is too small.' Never before had it had so much meaning: this *had* to be Derek's new beginning.

But of course what I was really craving wasn't just words but the emotion, personality, the essence of the man I loved. I thought I had seen a flicker of that sometimes on FaceTime, particularly when the children were talking to him and he almost seemed to be smiling, a strange crooked smile. It wasn't a smile we had ever seen before but the children especially were convinced it was there.

His mum thought so too. 'I swear he was smiling last night when his dad was mucking about and I told him off – you know, like I always tell Ken off,' she reported to me proudly. 'He looked like he was almost laughing, although it could have been a cough.' He was still occasionally struggling with his breathing, but then again his mum having a go at his dad always made him chuckle so, as ever, it could have been either.

He began to get more and more movement on his right side, but sometimes he couldn't stop it. He would move his fingers on his good hand, his right hand, to grab or squeeze something that had been placed in it – a bobbly plastic ball or a soft piece of fabric, things the team thought might stimulate sensation – and then he couldn't stop. He would squeeze and squeeze and squeeze until eventually it had to be taken away. This, they explained, was called perseverance. It meant he had a signal to do something but could not initiate the off switch, so it carried on and on in a constant loop between his brain and his fingers. Sometimes it was disturbing to see, because it looked so alien, so unlike him. But I tried to think of it as progress. Surely more movement meant it was likely there would be even more?

I was constantly trying to think of new ways to stimulate him. I knew how much he loved our garden, and had even FaceTimed him from it, showing him how everything was blossoming. He had been in a hermetically sealed hospital room for months and months. The windows couldn't be opened for safety reasons so he had had no fresh air, felt no breeze on his skin, seen no rain on the back of his hand. I thought bringing some nature to him might help to connect him to the world outside his alien interior one. I brought in a pot plant and some of his favourite reeds from the garden along with the heads of large ornamental daisies. I put the reed into his good hand and closed his fingers over it, saying, 'Here, feel your favourite reeds, feel the life force in them.' I know it sounds a bit hippie but I believe there is a life force that flows through all living things and I wanted him to have some of it.

'They've grown enormously this year,' I told him. 'Some are six foot high … you won't believe it when you see them!

I can't wait for you to come home and sit in your favourite chair in the garden and watch them rustle in the breeze.'

He looked at me, then down to the leaf in his fingers, started stroking it and feeling it between finger and thumb, again and again, then harder, then in a frenzy. The leaf started to shred, to fall apart, bits flying on to the floor. It was in equal parts inspiring and disturbing to see this little outburst. I could see the intention, the determination in him – he couldn't stop.

'You want that life force, don't you?' I said to him softly.

He looked me hard in the eye.

'Well, you have it. You are amazing, *amazing.*'

He looked back at his hand. There was nothing left in it, and he had stopped moving his fingers. He had managed to turn off the signal. More progress.

My friend June, a healer, had been telling me that in her view the body has to heal first before the mind can. The physical has to be conquered before the emotional. She believed that all of his healing energy had been going into keeping him alive, recovering enough basic function for the body to sustain itself.

'It's the natural instinct. Survival first, body second,' she told me.

It made sense in theory. My other healer friend, Gouri, who specializes in Reiki, said it was vital I gave him as much as possible a sense of love and security while he was in his frightening state. I didn't know anything about Reiki and had never tried it but she said that didn't matter because Derek believed in it. He'd had regular Reiki sessions when he was recovering from his breakdown and still went occasionally, for long after I'd got to know him. He even boasted that he had the power to Reiki-heal himself, having learnt from a Native American friend in the US.

Who knew if Derek actually did have the power to heal, but Gouri said that the fact he was open to it at the very least would be helpful. She taught me how to channel some healing energy. She suggested that I hover my hand over the top of his head and say, 'You are connected to the universe, to a life force beyond your control. Be free to open and connect.' And to keep repeating it. Then I was to do the same, but hovering my hand over his third eye, a spot believed to be in the middle of the forehead. This time I had to say, 'You are safe, you are loved. You are safe, you are loved, you are worthy.' Then finally I was to put my hands over his heart and simply repeat softly, 'Love, love, love …' over and over again.

I was watching my hands, making sure I didn't touch his chest as I knew it wasn't allowed as he still had various tubes connected and it might even scare him. Then I looked back at his face and, to my surprise, he was looking directly at me. And were my eyes deceiving me or was he also mouthing 'Love'? Tiny movements of the lips, but still there. I pulled my mask down so he could see my lips move and again kept saying, 'Love, love, love,' over and over again, looking straight at him.

Yes! It was unmistakable! He made no sound, but it was much clearer now that he was saying it too.

'Oh my God, he's saying "love" back,' came a voice from

behind me. A nurse had come into the room and was quietly standing in the corner. I hadn't noticed her, but she could see it too. It wasn't just me imagining things. I kept going, but after a little while longer he started to fade. His lips stopped moving, his eyes seemed to disconnect and he slipped away into unconsciousness.

But it had happened. That memory wasn't going to slip away from me.

Afterwards I discussed it with a neuropsychologist. Was it real? Did he mean 'love'? Was he trying to communicate with me? Did he understand love? Did he know I loved him and was trying to give it to him? He said it was hard to tell, while staying grounded in science. It might be that he did – or again, it could just have been that he was copying my lip movements, experimenting with control of his lips. After all, chimps in the zoo will try to pull their lips back in a smile to their keepers when they are smiled at, even though the equivalent expression in chimp language is an aggressive tactic. They are just doing it to try to relate to their keepers. *Exactly!* I thought, seeing the positive as ever.

'He might not remember me, might not love me, might not even know who I am – but he's trying to connect, and that's a start. It could be a new connection, a new bond!' I said to him. 'And who knows? He might be feeling love too,' I added for good measure. If you can't prove he isn't, I thought, I'm going to run with it. Hope.

Nevertheless, I had still seen no emotion or any real sign that he could feel. Even the mouthing of 'love' had been delivered with a frozen, flat, empty expression. And as time passed and I couldn't get him to repeat the word, either on a visit or FaceTime, my confidence was hard to maintain. If the nurse hadn't also witnessed it I would have started to doubt myself.

Then, one day on FaceTime I was talking 'at' him, looking straight into his eyes. It's an odd thing, isn't it, video contact? Many of us have experienced it with Zoom calls for work. In normal communication you aren't constantly staring. You're looking down at your notes in a meeting or at your food if you are sharing a meal, or you're looking around you. Not staring hard into people's eyes. At home Derek and I wouldn't stare at each other all the time. We were busy doing other things – eating, loading the dishwasher, lying in bed chatting, but not locked into that hard stare. It was unnatural. And as I chatted to him it reminded me of that second date, when he had forced me to dance to Aerosmith's 'I Don't Want To Miss A Thing' and I had squirmed and tried to release myself from his gaze.

As I stared into that iPad screen I said to him, 'This reminds me of that date – do you remember it? – when you forced me to stare into your eyes? I kept trying to look away but you wouldn't let me.' I carried on chatting about it, then asked him directly, 'Do you remember?' And his face started to crumple and contort in a strange way.

'Don't worry!' I said. 'It doesn't matter if you don't.'

I was concerned that I was somehow distressing him, that I would give him a seizure. But his face continued to crumple and I suddenly realized he was crying, actual tears streaming down his cheeks. Oh God, had I upset him? Was he scared or frustrated because he couldn't remember?

'*Do* you remember?' I asked again. To which he nodded. He actually nodded!

'You do! You do!' I yelped.

'Yes,' he mouthed. 'Yes … yes.' Then, to top it off, 'Of course,' as clear as a bell.

He *was* in there! He knew me!

I told him he was amazing, that he was a miracle, that it was all going to be OK, to which he sobbed and sobbed.

'I'm going to save you,' I said. 'I'm going to get you out, I promise.'

He stared at me … Again he was going, slipping back into unconsciousness. But he had come up from that deep ocean, for a minute, for a moment. So I knew it could happen again. The psychologists might have a scientific explanation for why it might not be 'real' but I knew in my gut it was, and it changed everything.

Chapter 12

Rebuild

_____

After that magical moment of recognition there were several further times when Derek would bob up from what I saw as his deep ocean of unconsciousness, and I would sense more connection with each one. More words were coming, all in whispers and used correctly. Each time he came up, I would try to fill him with as much belief as I could that he was going to get better. I would tell him to focus on the rehab, to try as hard as he could, that the better he got, the quicker he could come home. Home was his safe place, where he was loved and in control. It was a world away from where he was now: alone, frightened, unable to control his mind and body. He seemed to respond to this, and to latch on to home as hope, a way to have his life back.

However, at times it reached the point where I worried that he had focused on the idea of coming home as a solution to everything, that he believed he would be able to walk through the door into a world where he wasn't damaged, wasn't paralysed, wasn't struggling. That the trauma of Covid would go away as if he'd woken from a bad dream. The doctors were worried he was fixating on it, too, that he didn't understand how bad he was, that in his moments of greater consciousness he was creating a fantasy that would never be. It was a risk, but I felt the alternative for him was to be sucked down without hope. What was wrong with giving him something to aim for, to work towards, to keep him moving forward?

I talked to the doctors about the reality of coming home. Clearly, it was impossible now as Derek needed twenty-four-hour intensive care. But what about the future? After all, I wasn't just considering *his* future, but the entire family's, and it was becoming increasingly obvious that the children and I couldn't continue to live as we were. In our minds, we were still in a sort of suspended animation, where we had been since the moment Derek had got into that ambulance. Yes, I had gone back to work, and the children were back in schooling, but we were still mentally in waiting mode, holding on for the old Derek to return. We still had the *Welcome Home Daddy!* banners the kids had made in the first weeks after he went into hospital, when it had seemed impossible to believe he wouldn't be home before long, before we'd understood that it was possible he would die. They weren't pinned up on the wall, as I thought that would be too much like tempting Fate, but they were rolled up, waiting, albeit starting to crinkle and fade. A reminder of how much time had passed, and how dramatically Derek's story had changed.

His shoes were still by the front door, next to his wellies, as if he might come home at any minute to be helped into his favourite chair in the garden. We had had to keep alive the hope that *could* happen, but now we had to shift our expectations to meet what we could *make* happen in reality.

I took the *Field of Dreams* approach: if you build it, they will come. I chose a leap of faith: I would create a home in which Derek could be cared for, even if he remained as he was right now. That way, we were facing up to his changed self, and perhaps it would give us a base to hope for the future, safe home visits and maybe a move home. It might also help the kids and me to understand how our new relationship with Derek might evolve: me as wife *and* carer, Billy and Darcey as the children of a severely disabled dad.

There were practical challenges, of course, but even that side of it felt positive: whenever I threw myself into the practical, it helped me to manage my fears of whatever the future might bring. Derek and I had had plans to do certain things to the house once I was back from the jungle, and all year I had been thinking, Well, I can't do that now. This was partly because every bit of my limited focus was on Derek's health, on keeping him and our family going, but also because, like so many others with sick family members, we had been living at home in effective self-isolation, unable to have contractors and workmen in. Even if we had, at various points, been allowed to do so, it hadn't felt right.

But by autumn it wasn't a matter of waiting for lockdowns to end or Derek to get better that had held me back: I couldn't change anything aesthetic because I wanted Derek to be part of those choices, if possible, and I didn't want to do anything that might alter what he saw as home. I didn't want to render the place unrecognizable.

I was particularly aware of the impact his home environment might have on him because for months he had been entirely sealed off from the world. It wasn't just the closed windows and lack of nature, but the fact that everybody around him had been in full PPE: he'd seen only their eyes since the day he'd gone into the coma. When I'd visited him I'd had to wear a full mask, so he could only see my eyes too. Sometimes when I was sitting far away from him, so that we were more than two metres apart, I would just pull it down and mouth, 'I love you,' so he could see my mouth move. That he was trying to relearn how to speak yet never being permitted to see a mouth was heartbreaking. I know from having babies that your little one learns from facing you in the pram as you walk around, chatting to them absentmindedly: they watch every word.

No one was arguing that the necessary PPE situation wasn't putting his cognitive recovery at a massive disadvantage, so we started to talk about other ways to help him. By now he was off dialysis, had no tracheotomy, and was feeding through a tube in his stomach so that he had more of a chance to communicate and move around, even potentially for a short time out of the hospital. Perhaps we could ready him for home while we readied home for him.

Yes, it was going to be a big challenge. But it was also a practical mission that I could get my teeth into after so long hanging on dreams and manifestations. Derek was on a trajectory that was unknown in a world with no data for his condition, so having something solid to plan for felt like an anchor.

I discussed it with the hospital, who gave me an overview of the sort of changes I would need to make, but who also advised that this was a specialist field for a structural occupational therapist. We would have to wait months for one to come to us under the NHS, and the delay was likely to worsen with the pressure caused by Covid – already the waiting lists were frighteningly long. The other problem was that the NHS system for home preparation didn't activate until a hospital release date was confirmed and, of course, with Derek no one knew when or if ever he could be discharged.

The advice was to pay a private assessor, recommended by the hospital, to come now, in advance, to help us form a plan. It was money I didn't really have but, like everyone else, we'd had no holiday and were unlikely to for a long while. What better way to use any money we might have spent on going away to give the whole family a sense of the future? That was how I justified it to myself anyway.

The assessor was fantastic: she gave us some practical guidance but she was emotionally supportive too. She understood that my leap of faith that Derek would come home one day was vital for all of us to move forward. There were so many practicalities to tackle: first, like most semis, our bedroom and bathroom were on the first floor, not ground level. Stairs were clearly out of the question for Derek so we had to create 'one-floor living' for the whole family. That meant saying goodbye to our living room to make it into a bedroom, which in turn meant we had to extend the kitchen just enough to give us a family room that could incorporate a sofa and TV and space for a wheelchair or stretcher. The alternative was to put a lift up to the first floor, which was extremely expensive and impossible to achieve without tearing down half the house and effectively rebuilding it.

We also had to dismantle Derek's man cave, our old garage, which was attached to the house but, because it had been built in the 1930s, was too narrow for a modern car. He had long used it as a shed. Luckily it had a little loo at the back so plumbing was already built in. Now it could be turned into a wetroom for Derek. He had loved that garage, pottering in there at the weekends, and it was sad that we'd have to get rid of the space where Derek used to mend toys and do DIY: I felt as if I was giving up on something big Derek loved. But the reality was that, right now, he couldn't hold a hammer and I just had to stay in the practical. Stay on goal.

The other major consideration was making sure that doorways were widened enough for a wheelchair or stretcher to go through. We already knew that the house was unsuitable for such because Derek had broken his foot two or three years before and had had to use a wheelchair for six weeks. There were still great gashes in the doorframes where he had wedged himself on his way to make a cup of tea. The experience had brought home the daily challenges of living with a disability. I remember him saying, 'This is a nightmare. I can balance myself enough to put the kettle on but I can't pour the water in, and even if I could, I can't hold the mug and move myself, so I have to drink the tea by the kettle, rather than wheel myself back to my desk to sip where I'm working.' Of course, his challenge back then had simply been a non-weight-bearing foot. He'd still had strength and capacity elsewhere in his body and, most importantly, a fully conscious working brain to resolve the problems.

While I was wrangling with these practicalities, having conversations that would normally have been Derek's terrain, it still seemed he was desperate to get home, and this was more obvious every time he rose from that ocean of unconsciousness. It was as if he was pulling himself up on a rope that would lead him home, and I was hanging over the edge of a lifeboat holding on to him. He would bob up seemingly more aware, but would sink down again, staring, lost, sometimes for days. Every time he came up, I wanted to fill him with enough hope so that when he went back down he didn't give up. I had to keep encouraging him, giving him strength to cling to the rope that led to home and life.

As well as making changes that would make our home liveable for someone in Derek's state, I also wanted to give him the chance to experience what he loved about our home. We live on the side of a hill, so he could be wheeled into the front of the house relatively easily, but to go out of the back and into the garden had always meant a climb down some rickety steps: Derek's beloved garden would be inaccessible to him without an expensive lift. I compromised:

I'd prepare the foundations for a lift, trying to get as much of the disruptive work done before there was any hint of a return home, and put in glass patio doors.

For so long I had been visualizing and manifesting the idea of Derek sitting on our lawn enjoying the garden we loved so much, but that dream was still a good way off. I had spent hours picturing him sitting in the spot he called Tuscany, in his favourite chair, laughing and joking and accidentally getting sunburnt, as he did every time, then blaming me for not telling him to wear sunscreen, even though I had reminded him twenty times. I had tried night after night to make that scene alive and visual, and now I was realizing that the manifestations I'd made months ago would perhaps never happen.

Was I prepared to give up on Derek's garden dream? I think you know the answer to that … Changing the garden doors had been a goal of ours since we'd moved into the house. When we were deciding whether or not I should go into the jungle, I'd made myself feel better about being away from home for a month by resolving to use the money I was paid to get us big glass doors when I returned. We had joked as I left that as I lay in that place with bugs crawling all over me, I'd be saying to myself, Think of the glass doors, think of those sliding patio doors.

Instead I decided to combine two dreams. I imagined us sitting there in the morning, bathed in sunlight from our enormous new glass doors. At last we'd be able to see the garden and the sky as the sun rose and set. The children and I even imagined where Derek might sit or lie in the new room, and planted loads of bulbs where his eyeline might be, visualizing him seeing them and being inspired by new life, new home. It helped me to feel that the building works were practical, to make it easier for him to come home as his new self, *and* that they would fulfil our long-held dreams. Everything had been put on hold for so long: the children's dreams, career dreams, holiday dreams, the lot. It was time to let those dreams in again. And I thought, If Derek gets a little bit better and can use a wheelchair, then at least he can sit and see the garden. And the next stage, if there is a progression, can be putting in the lift. Somehow. Some day.

I threw myself into the project, and tried to embrace the massive disruption it caused at home. Building works are never fun while they're going on, with all of the mess and chaos they entail, but at least I could try to manage the renovations alongside visiting Derek. I was able, for instance, to take some tiles intended for his new wetroom to show him. I hope it helped him to feel involved and to understand more how I was trying to help him progress.

But it wasn't plain sailing. I had set myself Christmas as a finish date, not because I had ever realistically believed he would be home for good by then, but because I felt that if I could at least make our home a clean and quiet environment for the children, ready for whatever the festive season might hold, 2021 might bring us a fresh start, a chance to get back to normal. We were hearing announcements that a vaccine being developed would be available sooner than originally expected so it might be possible to start the year ready and prepared for Derek's best-case scenario.

But then talk of lockdowns returned, and as the new variants and their increased rate of infection spread, more and more people around us were getting sick, and the reality of Covid started to make itself known even to those who had been lucky enough to escape the first wave. The workmen digging the lift foundations outside fell ill and rightly took weeks off to isolate. Delays kept coming, and the novelty of effectively 'camping' in their own home had long worn off for the children.

Was I creating a world of chaos for my family to prepare for something that was never going to happen? Were these the same optimistic delusions that had led me down blind alleys in the past? Like the times I had kept planning romantic weekends away with boyfriends who had long since stopped loving me? Then came the return of national lockdown, and with it renewed doubt about a brighter future and a better new year, and whether it might be available to any of us.

As with so many families, Christmas is an essential part of our year. And for us it was neither Santa, nor gifts, nor fancy meals that made the season, but being together as a family. Which meant that Derek was a fundamental part of every moment. We always spent Christmas Eve and Christmas Day in Chorley with his family, and even our journey up there was always a fun part of our festive ritual. Derek would decorate the car with lights, load up the stereo with Christmas songs and we'd dress up and dress the kids in nativity costumes for the entire journey. It made even the slog of a long motorway drive feel like fun – an event!

– especially when Derek's fabric reindeer antlers buckled each time they hit the car roof.

I knew we wouldn't have any of that this year, as there would be no travelling up north anyway, but we had hoped that the rest of his family might be able to come down, somehow get the chance to see Derek and spend some time with him. And that he, the children and I might at least be together for some of the festive season. Sure, we wouldn't be making our traditional stop at our favourite service station en route to Chorley, all of us whooping with laughter as Derek got out in full costume to fill up the car, but we could have *something*, couldn't we?

But Christmas was causing pain for the whole country, and as the strain of living in a building site during the middle of winter mounted, I began to dread it. How would we cope without Derek, when he and his little rituals made it such a special season for us? Even buying the children's presents wasn't enough: although I had done that in the past, it had always been Derek who had found the little extras, the gifts we would still be talking about as spring came round, the magic dust that made Christmas. As anxiety gave way to panic attacks, I tried to remind myself that the workmen and I were not just trying to get some building work finished by Christmas, but were hacking a path to our future, to *all* the Christmases we might yet have.

News reports increasingly discussed whether the entire Christmas season was in jeopardy, the promised five-day amnesty collapsing as the infection and hospitalization numbers rocketed. Things seemed to change hour by hour as the lockdown tier system kept being adjusted, and there was understandable anger that the festivals of non-Christian worshippers had effectively been cancelled at a moment's notice while the national preoccupation with Christmas continued. But I could see that Christmas was always bigger than religion: it marks the end of something and takes place at the time of the solstice too. Long before Christianity, the pagans had held their own festivals, lighting fires to encourage the sun to return. They knew they needed something in the depths of a long dark winter to help them believe that the days would grow longer and that the land would warm again.

The worse the news got, the more the national mood seemed to be that the country needed Christmas more than ever to keep everyone going into an increasingly bleak-looking new year. And so did Derek. His spirit was failing. He was showing signs of almost wanting to give up. I *had* to give him something to believe in, even if that was just us being ready for him at Christmas, regardless of whether he could come home yet.

As the date drew closer, it became apparent that the renovation project would come down to the wire – if Derek was going to make it home at all. Nothing was finished. We were all camped in my bedroom as the rest of the house was covered with builders' dust. We were all fed up with it, but knew we were doing it so that Dad could come home one day. And then the house flooded. The work they were doing for the wetroom, the builders' equipment, Billy's toys, all of our Christmas presents – everything was soaked.

I wondered if I was now just one of those people to whom terrible things happen. I was not so much exhausted by the events than by having nothing but bad news to share. I felt as if a part of me had been taken away by all of this: the cheeriness, the positivity, the ability to action my way out of a crisis – it was starting to fade.

But the only thing we could do was to carry on. The next day the hospital sent a specialist bed. The man delivering it stood at the doorstep and said bluntly, 'I can't come in because of Covid so you've got to put it together yourself.'

Twenty minutes later I was sitting in what had been our front room, where Derek would regale people at dinner parties with stories of political intrigue, where we had family movie nights, where I'd played with my babies. I was there, plonked on the floor of this room that had been stripped of furniture to make space for equipment, with this guy at the window telling me how to set the bed up. My shoulders slumped as I thought, How come I'm putting together a hospital bed not to help a friend, or for an elderly relative, but for my husband because he may never get out of bed? What could I do but plough on?

Just as it seemed that this scene couldn't be more piti-ful, the children came in. I was worried that seeing such evidence of Dad's current tragic state might frighten them, might make the relationship they'd had with him seem even fainter. But they seemed almost excited. They wanted to go through all the equipment and try it out, having a proper laugh at the hydraulics on the bed. And as I watched them goofing about, I realized that the reality was bringing them closer to what their future with their dad was going to look like, and actually making it less fearful. Laughing about it neutered some of the pain. I felt proud to have put that bed together, even at my lowest ebb. It felt like trying to normalize our new life. If you come home from school, and suddenly see a hospital bed where your dad is now going to sleep, and strange equipment taking up half the house, of *course* you'll be anxious about who is coming home one day. I let them play on it as much as they wanted, so it was lovely to see their ease with it.

Then came Boris Johnson's announcement just days before 25 December, which changed everything. Now we knew that no one would have the time with their loved ones they had planned for, and we realized the new year would be far from normal. I assumed any chance of visiting Derek would be cancelled, and prepared the children for the worst. After ten months of waiting, it was unbearable for them that they might not get to see their dad, and I suspect the hospital knew this. So I will always be grateful they managed to allow us the time together that they did.

The moment the children first saw him was magical. Billy was in floods of tears immediately and, ignoring all previous warnings not to get close to Derek because of social distancing, couldn't stop himself rushing forward for a hug. Darcey characteristically tried to hold herself back a bit, to do the right thing ... until she couldn't wait any longer.

He was there with them, really there. You could see the wonder and delight in all their eyes. Of course he was hugely changed, but they seemed able to look past that, and to focus on the obvious love flowing between them. They adapted to the changes so fast and with such huge hearts that I was bursting with pride for all three of them. Derek was weak, paralysed, and not his full self. But his spirit was there. I was certain he knew who he was and who we were, and that he knew it was Christmas. We played a version of charades, and Billy showed him the Lego things they had effectively built 'together', back when Billy had been on FaceTime with Derek 'watching' from his hospital bed. They had spent hours like this, just as Darcey had while she had been making all of the furniture for her bedroom. 'This is the one Susanna Reid sent to us,' Billy explained, 'back when you were first ill, Dad, and we were all so worried you were going to die.' It was as if they were somehow filling him in on stuff they hadn't been able to share with him – and Derek appeared to be taking it in. I was watching a gap closing.

'I'll be back soon,' I whispered to him, as I got up to head home. 'This is just the beginning.' And I meant it.

But within a couple of days we were back into national lockdown, unable to visit each other at all. Suddenly, instead of Covid being something that had all but faded from the national consciousness, it seemed everyone knew someone who was seriously sick. 'Long Covid' was by now part of the virus lexicon and, like the virus itself, was developing more and more variants. Even those who had never been hospitalized were now discovering, months on, there was damage throughout their bodies. It was a winter longer than any of us could have imagined while we were 'eating out to help out' in those summer days, or being told that returning to the office was our civic duty.

And now here we are in spring. The bulbs we planted back in the autumn as we hoped that Derek might one day come home are up and blooming. A sign of the force of nature, fighting back after months of winter. It's so inspiring, so reassuring, and it's also a reminder that it is now more than a year since Covid tore Derek from us. Without the chance to visit him in person, to lift him up from that deep ocean of unconsciousness, the doctors and I can see that he has slipped back, now able only to nod or to give one-word whispers at best. It's as if he has disengaged, disheartened by the size of the task in hand. The promise of home and a future life still seem so far away.

But hasn't that been the case for all of us to some degree? In the first few desperate months of this year, as the news came that cases and deaths were higher than ever, it felt as if the entire nation slumped into a weary sadness that none of us had experienced last spring when all of this was a terrifying novelty. Now all of us, including Derek, have struggled to find any sense of hope at all.

But with true hope you have to know that nothing can truly quash it. We just have to hold on to it for a little longer, a little harder, and to look for signs that our futures haven't been lost and are just waiting to be renewed once more. The vaccine rollout is no magic bullet but it is a beacon of hope that the most vulnerable will be protected and the rest of us can start to rebuild: to regenerate our livelihoods, our relationships, and to see an end to the torture of loneliness and isolation. For Derek hope is still there too. I will fight on, at least knowing that I have done it before, so I can do it again. There are new treatments on the horizon, signs that we may be able to see him in person, to hold out that lifeline to haul him back soon. He is still alive. And so is hope.

Epilogue

When I started writing this book, I imagined that by the time you came to read the paperback I would be reminding you of long-past horrors. It seemed out of the question that we might still be feeling the repercussions when the paperback came around. Back then, all of us, as much as we could predict anything at all, assumed that two years on we would be in a much happier place, where Covid was a fading memory, the crisis largely forgotten. Instead, that clear threshold we hoped to cross, when things would be 'back to normal', has not quite made itself clear. And for many of us it has been easy to feel left behind, to feel as if we haven't crossed the threshold at all.

For most of 2020, I dared not look beyond a single day. But if I had, I would have assumed that by now, if Derek were to survive, our lives would be back to the familiar routines of work, school and play. Mercifully he *is* alive, and he is now home with us, but our world is so very far from the way it was before.

Isn't that the same for all of us, though? Aren't we all having to learn a new way of life, with different considerations, different economics, even different global politics? For a split second, in the pub or the café, we can forget how much has shifted. But for those who were caught in the eye of the storm, it really is only a split second. Yes, we have the vaccines. Yes, we can now go to a football match, a gig, a wedding – but these are never quite what they were before. We are more anxious. We are still grieving. We are still getting back on our feet. Or we are simply still going through a process of necessary adjustment.

I think there are a lot of people who have felt forgotten as the world has started to open up. Maybe you are one of them. Maybe you still are suffering the direct health effects of Covid yourself, or are feeling the loss of a loved one, or your own vital health appointments have been delayed, your income depleted or your mental health impacted. There are legions of us still feeling far from what we were. This means that some days it is hard to hear 'Isn't it great, life getting back to normal?' when what you're feeling is 'I'm not normal! My business is going under. My Mum's gone. My mental health is suffering.'

Too much has changed: we have seen too much, we have been through too much, we have learnt too much, as individuals, as a community and as a nation. There will be so much we want to forget, to wipe away: the pain of loss, the destruction of livelihoods, the separation, the loneliness, the fear.

So if that is you, know that you're not forgotten. We ~~are~~ united. We will keep going – we'll keep the hope, and we'll bring the joy back.

We must grieve for those things we have lost, but as we pick ourselves up and face our new future, wouldn't it be wonderful if we could keep some of the pockets of joy that have sustained us through these darkest of times? To hang on to the community spirit, the waves of kindness, the urge to do something for the greater good. As we emerge into our new lives, wouldn't it be great if we could let hope lead us to new opportunities, and a new confidence in how we can cope with hardship?

Before the Covid crisis, I think most of us assumed that the world we lived in was relatively safe. We didn't have to think about how risky our lives were every minute of every day. I know I certainly didn't. I would get into a car and drive, focused on getting from A to B, not thinking about the statistics of road accidents with every turn of the wheel. Those statistics aren't broadcast in the way the Covid death rates have been and still are, but of course the lives lost are just as devastating for the individuals affected. It was easier to hide from how uncertain and frightening our world has always been, and how things can change when we least expect them to. But because with the pandemic we have all faced the same threat at the same time, we have become painfully aware of how uncertain life is.

On top of this is the fact that the things we *were* afraid of before haven't gone away. The environmental crisis and global warming are more frightening than ever, their impact encroaching ever closer. The bills still need to be paid, no one has found a money tree. The diseases, health worries and

...ns about our own lives and those of our loved
... there. Covid may have knocked these out of
... s, but of course it hasn't wiped them away. They
... king in the shadows, ready to spring back out at
us as ... as we're no longer caught in the Covid headlights.

But we can't let fear dominate our future. We can't spend
every day imagining that the worst will happen, just because
some of the worst predictions of Covid *did*. Rather, we must
go forward together with a renewed sense of what matters
to us most: we must be more conscious than ever of not
taking anything for granted, and of expressing gratitude for
what and whom we love.

It is still a daily struggle for me to adjust to my changed
and still changing life. I have learnt to live with uncertainty,
like so many of us have had to. While I know Derek's health
is still fragile, I also know that he's still here, and that gives me
courage to fight on, to tackle the challenges of where Derek
is now and what the future may hold for him and our family.

I got the moment that I once longed for, the miracle of him
coming home, and for that I am truly grateful. But our life
is far from what it was before. How could it be? Derek can't
move for himself, he has no conversation, words are mouthed
in whispers, one or two at a time, and he often sleeps twenty
out of twenty-four hours a day. And we still have no guarantees that this can ever change. The Derek who has come
home is very different from the man who left, just as our old
lives and the freedoms we longed for during that first lockdown now seem changed, maybe even lost for ever.

But does that mean that the hope that sustained me

through last year was futile? Not at all. I believe in the true power of hope more than ever. However dark some days might still be, when I feel alone and lost it's always there, like an internal battery keeping me driving forward.

I see hope's power in the miracle that Derek has survived at all, and in the miracle that the scientists have developed vaccines and treatments that have saved so many of us. I see it in the way Derek tries to be a husband to me and a dad to Darcey and Billy. He might not be able to communicate in a way that most people could understand, but he increasingly mouths words, phrases even, that are so very *him*. And we have had magical moments, such as finally getting him down into the garden, to sit 'in Tuscany' as he used to call it, and where I used to dream of seeing him again.

Of course, his enjoyment of it is very different now. He can't run around building assault courses for the kids or bellowing his latest opinions at us all. But he is finding a new way to show us his love: flickers of the eyes, smiles at the kids, fun and games. Long, wide-eyed gazes at the beauty of an evening sky, the wonder of nature around him. And we as a family are finding new ways of loving him back and loving our lives together.

Yet to me, the true power of hope is not just holding on to the wish that Derek can recover more, as forceful as that might be. Only doing that would be missing the point. Because it isn't about focusing on the lack of something, wanting that gap to be filled, or about going back to the way things were before, when we thought we were happy. And nor is it about jumping forward to what we think will be our happy future. Hope isn't about wishing for things to be perfect, but about finding a way of accepting that while something may not be perfect, there are still infinite ways we can work, love and thrive within it.

So now, when I'm tending to Derek's feed or medication, or helping him to stretch his limbs, I try to see the beauty in the new intimacy we have. It doesn't have to be grim, it doesn't have to be the worst thing imaginable. That is something which anybody who is caring for someone who is sick or vulnerable knows. And suddenly the fear of it eases. Just as some things appall us before we have children (A messy house! A broken ornament! A dirty nappy!), we adapt without thinking, and we do it with an open heart. In many ways, our slow modification of everyday life is very similar.

I won't be consumed by the tragedy in the situation and I don't want that for our family. We need to laugh, we need to find joy through it all. And I don't want to live a life defined by what has happened – even if every part of our everyday life is now affected by it.

Hope is not a desire, a longing for something that means we've failed if we don't achieve it. It's the belief that you can get through anything with love, standing shoulder to shoulder with people and looking forward. Hope is holding on to these things, even when you feel that the darkness will never lift. Because when tomorrow comes, which it will, it may not be just the world that has changed, but you. You could have shifted how you see the world, redefined what you want from it.

Hope is real, and it's the best way forward to find your own wonderful future.

Acknowledgements

I have been struggling to write proper acknowledgements to thank all the people who have made this book possible. My problem is that the list is longer than the book itself. It includes every single one of my family, the Drapers and the Garraways, every friend, colleague, health worker, and every person who holds Derek dear. And also every stranger who has reached out with a kind word or action. You have all kept me going, kept me feeling that the pain of writing my own personal tale in the ongoing horror story we have all been living is worth it, that reading it might help you. I trust you will all know how grateful I am.

So I am going to keep my thanks here specific to the production of the book itself. To everyone at Transworld, particularly Michelle Signore and Susanna Wadeson for their determination to see this through and for their huge patience, along with the brilliant Alex Heminsley for helping me find the right words when I struggled to. You are amazing. Also Hazel Orme, Mari Roberts, Kate Samano, Katrina Whone and Eleanor Updegraff in the editorial team, Richard Ogle and Graeme Andrew in design, photographer Pål Hansen, production director Cat Hillerton, Becky Short in publicity and Josh Crosley in the rights team. Eternal thanks to Matt Nicholls, Zoe Ross and all at United Agents for their support and love, which no commission could ever reward. And to Max Dundas and James Delamare for their wisdom, guidance and endless disrupted weekends.

To all at ITV for their support and continued 'being there', particularly Neil Thompson, Emma Gormley and Katie Rawcliffe. To Ashley Tabor at Global Radio, whose generosity of support has so moved me, and to James Daniels, my Smooth Radio producer, whose patience and brilliance are an inspiration. Thank you to Mary, Jackie, Tommy and Sarah for their ceaseless friendship and support. Thanks to Piers Morgan for convincing me that I had the strength to write this book in the first place, and to Global's John Chittenden for virtually standing over me with love and builder's tea, saying, 'Stop staring into space and just write!' Thank you to David Morgan, Caroline and Gouri Lai for all your wisdom. And lastly and most importantly to Derek, Darcey and Billy, who every day show me the true Power of Hope.

Kate Garraway is a British television and radio presenter and journalist. She began working in television in 1994, when she joined the south edition of ITV News Central as a production journalist, reporter and news presenter. Kate has worked on *ITV News Meridian*, *Sunrise* on Sky News, *GMTV* and *Daybreak*, which in 2014 was replaced by *Good Morning Britain*. Kate currently presents alongside Ben Shepherd, Susanna Reid and Piers Morgan. Kate came fourth in 2019's *I'm a Celebrity . . . Get Me Out of Here!* and also appeared in the fifth series of *Strictly Come Dancing* with professional partner Anton du Beke.